"Many women are now realizing that the span of time surrounding menopause is much more than a medically defined continuum of change within a woman's reproductive system. We are discovering together that, for us, it is a life passage that needs to be recognized as such and honored by moving it from a passive state to an active state. . . . As we choose actively to engage in changing, we experience a transformation of life energy. We can rename our experience, choosing to discover our bodies as life-giving and thus sacred, connecting us with the Divine."

— *Drawing from the Women's Well*, pp. 23–24

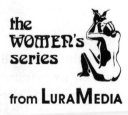

the
WOMEN's
series

from LuraMedia

What women are saying about
Drawing from the Women's Well...

This is a book of affirmation, of power, and of wisdom. It affirms the power and dignity of the life passage of menopause . . . it probes the wisdom at the center of women's lives in such a manner that all who read and ponder it can live more fully into the second half of female knowing, grieving, and re-creating. . . . A splendid contribution.
> — Maria Harris, author, *Dance of the Spirit:*
> *The Seven Steps of Women's Spirituality*

A joyful invitation to gather with our elders who are coming to view on the other side of menopause.
> — Marjory Zoet Bankson, President, Faith at Work;
> author, *Braided Streams* and *Seasons of Friendship*

Joan Borton's book enables women to experience the passage to the latter decades of life as a time of discovery, of new friendships, or re-discovered gifts. It liberates women from lingering shame, from the culturally imposed feeling that to enter the "infertile" years is to become a leftover, less than a woman. Women together are discovering delight, wisdom, and energy through and beyond menopause, supporting each other in searching and grieving and renewing. This book will given women courage in their search and a sense of peaceful purpose.
> — Rosemary Haughton, author, lecturer, member of Wellspring Home,
> Gloucester, Massachusetts

Reading this book is like being wrapped in a grandmother's quilt of women's wisdom. I highly recommend it.
> — Christiane Northrup, M.D.; FACOG; Assistant Clinical
> Professor of Ob-Gyn, University of Vermont, College of Medicine

Joan Borton shows us our connection to the sacred female essence.
> — Sadja Greenwood, M.D.; author, *Menopause, Naturally*;
> Assistant Clinical Professor, University of California, San Francisco

An important and empowering look at one woman's process of reclaiming menopause from the stereotypical and mythical. In sharing so extensively from her own journal writings, Ms. Borton provides all women with a model for integrating menopause — physiologically, psychologically, and spiritually — into their own life histories. DRAWING FROM THE WOMEN'S WELL affirms the importance to women of all phases of their reproductive lives and the opportunity provided by menopause for remembering and releasing past modes of power and relationship and learning new forms.
> — Meg Clark, Ph.D., Behavioral Sciences Department,
> California State Polytechnic University

A book that goes far beyond menopause, reflecting on all life passages . . . and their potential for growth.
> — Anne C. Brower, M.D., Professor of Radiology and Nuclear Medicine,
> Uniformed Services University of the Health Sciences, Bethesda, Maryland

A book that will decrease fear and increase self-esteem and appreciation of women's experiences as we take our rightful place in the circle of elders. . . . A unique and creative complement to other materials on this important time of transition . . . concentrating on women's feelings, choices and cycles, and spiritual connections.
> — Diana Laskin Siegal, co-author, *Ourselves, Growing Older:*
> *Women Aging with Knowledge and Power*

Drawing
from the
Women's Well

Reflections on the Life Passage of Menopause

JOAN C. BORTON

San Diego, California

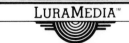

LURAMEDIA™

LuraMedia
7060 Miramar Road, Suite 104
San Diego, CA 92121

Library of Congress Cataloging-in-Publication Data

Borton, Joan C., date
    Drawing from the women's well : reflections on the life passage of
menopause / by Joan C. Borton.
        p.   cm. — (The Women's series)
    Includes bibliographical references.
    ISBN 0-931055-87-3
    1. Menopause—Psychological aspects.   I. Title.   II. Series:
Women's series (San Diego, Calif.)
RG186.B67   1992
612.6'65—dc20   91-45192
                                                        CIP

For Mary,
my mother

Grateful acknowledgment is made to the following copyright holders for permission to use their copyrighted material:

Bantam Books, a division of Bantam, Doubleday, Dell Publishing Group, Inc., for the quotation from *Dance of the Spirit: Seven Steps of Women's Spirituality*, by Maria Harris. Copyright 1989 by Maria Harris. Used by permission.

Bantam Books, a division of Bantam, Doubleday, Dell Publishing Group, Inc., for the quotation from *Focusing*, by Eugene T. Gendlin. Copyright 1981. Used by permission.

Beacon Press, for quotations from *The Sacred Hoop: Recovering the Feminine in American Indian Traditions*, by Paula Gunn Allen. Copyright 1986 by Paula Gunn Allen. Used by permission.

Beacon Press, for the quotation from *Diving Deep and Surfacing: Women Writers on Spiritual Quest*, by Carol Christ. Copyright 1980 by Carol Christ. Used by permission.

Beacon Press, for quotations from *The Journey Is Home*, by Nelle Morton. Copyright 1985 by Nelle Morton. Used by permission.

Beacon Press, for quotations from *Lost Goddesses of Early Greece: A Collection of Pre-Hellenic Myths*, by Charlene Spretnak. Copyright 1984 by Charlene Spretnak. Used by permission.

Jean Shinoda Bolen, for the quotation from her lecture, "Women's Spirituality," Watertown, Massachusetts, January 1988. Used by permission.

The Crossroad Publishing Company, for quotations from *Journey Through Menopause: A Personal Rite of Passage*, by Christine Downing. Copyright 1987 by Christine Downing. Used by permission.

Doubleday, a division of Bantam, Doubleday, Dell Publishing Group, Inc., for quotations from *Lifesigns: Intimacy, Fecundity, and Ecstasy in Christian Perspective*, by Henri J. M. Nouwen. Copyright 1986 by Henri J. M. Nouwen. Used by permission.

Fawcett-Columbine, Ballentine Books, for the quotation from *The Goddess Within*, by Jennifer Barker Woolger and Roger J. Woolger. Copyright 1989 by Jennifer Barker Woolger and Roger J. Woolger. Used by permission of Random House, Inc.

Firebrand Books, Ithaca, New York, for quotations from *Getting Home Alive*, by Aurora Levins Morales and Rosario Morales. Copyright 1986 by Aurora Levins Morales and Rosario Morales. Used by permission.

Betty Friedan, for the quotation from her speech "Real Choices: A New Feminine Mystique," Smith College, June 1990. Used by permission.

Stewart, Tabori & Chang, Inc., for quotations from *I Dream a World: Portraits of Black Women Who Changed America*, by Brian Lanker (Stewart, Tabori & Chang, 1989). Used with permission of the publisher.

Thames and Hudson, Inc., for the quotation from *Celtic Mysteries: The Ancient Religion*, by John Sharkey. Copyright © 1987 by Thames and Hudson. Reprinted by permission of the publisher.

Wellesley College, Wellesley, Massachusetts, The Stone Center for Development Services and Studies, for quotations from "From Depression to Sadness in Women's Psychotherapy," by Irene P. Stiver and Jean Baker Miller. *Work in Progress*, No. 36, 1988. Used by permission.

Wellesley College, Wellesley, Massachusetts, The Stone Center for Development Services and Studies, for the quotation from "The Mother-Daughter Relationship: Themes in Psychotherapy," a tape by Janet Surrey, 1989. Used by permission.

Woman of Power, for the quotation from "Menopause: A Journey Homeward," by Connie Batten. Copyright 1989 by *Woman of Power*. Used by permission.

Contents

Acknowledgments

I am grateful for the encouragement of my family:

- my husband, Cam, who has believed in me, shared my excitement, and been there when I wanted to give up;
- my children — Jenni, Lawrie, and Jim — whose appreciation and enthusiasm about this project have helped to carry me;
- my mother, Mary, whose thoughtful and diligent readings of each chapter have yielded many helpful suggestions;
- my father, Ross, who has had an eye for material relevant to my project. His findings have often stimulated my thought.

I doubt that I would have completed this book without the skillful coaching of Kathleen Spivack. My enjoyment of the process increased through the working relationship with my editor, Nancy Hardesty.

I thank Andy Canale for posing the question: "Why wait?" and for his excitement about the writing process.

I am indebted to and have been supported by the women who have shared their experience with me: "The Research Group," whose support for this project was immediate and wholehearted: Wendy, Suzanne, Nancy, Gloria, Jan, and Sheilagh. I have received from them and others who have been willing to explore this life passage with me. I am grateful to the women who have put their experience into words expressing their discoveries: Liz, Nancy, Babette, Jeanne, Martha, Maureen, Petie, Linda, Rebecca, Deane, Carole, Diana, Nancy Jo, Sue, Lynn, Cynthia, Cheryl, Jan, Jean, Barb, and Sandra.

To Joan and Tom who encouraged me to hold my vision and to those who shared their editorial and clerical gifts: Cayte, who helped me put my first thoughts about menopause into writing; Camilla, who has been my technical teacher; Sandy and Melody, who were there with support when I needed them, I say thank you.

Emery House has been a sacred place for me. There in the silence and rhythm of the daily office, I have been able to rest and write. I am grateful.

This writing project has been part of a harvest that has brought blessing into my life. I am deeply grateful to the Source and Giver of Life.

Preface

After ten years of curtailed activity as the result of a back injury, I was physically able at fifty-two to start mountain climbing again. Beginning with small hikes, I gained stamina. So it was with great joy and gratitude that I began the climb up a nearby mountain that I had looked at for thirty years and never climbed.

Walking steadily upward for two-and-a-half hours, I remembered the promise of water noted in the guide book. I was thirsty as I made my way along the narrow mountain path. Greenness was on either side and overhead. A cool wind blew through the hardwood trees. As I came into pines, spruce, and other evergreens, I saw a great rock beside the path. An arrow pointed to its base. Looking down, I saw a small pool of clear, mountain spring water coming up from a source deep beneath the boulder. Sensing the holiness of the moment and the place, I knelt down and reached with cupped hands to drink.

In the silence of that green cathedral, I knew within my being why springs and wells were once considered sacred. I understood why my Celtic forebears in Ireland made shrines at springs and built wells at these "womb-openings of the Earth Mother." Often these constructions have carvings in their stone of the Mother Goddess, pictured in her three forms. As Maiden, Mother, and Crone, the figures carry an infant, a cornucopia, and a basket of fruit.[1]

I remember seeing a picture of all three forms, each with a symbol of their phase of womanhood, carved into the stone of an ancient well. It was one of those holy wells and springs that "have been sacred from time immemorial. Despite outward changes in image or ritual, the act of invocation of the source of life has never wavered."[2] These holy wells or sacred centers were places for the thirsty pilgrim, like myself, to stop in gratitude for replenishment from the deep, life-giving Source, and they were often meeting places, the centers of village life.

In many cultures this sacred center has been a place of gathering and sharing for women. Although this is not true in our culture, the women's well has been a powerful symbol for me. My personal image of this reality has been a gift from my mother. In our home when I was a child, we had a brass water jug. It often prompted wonderful stories from my mother about village life in India, where she grew up as a missionary child. My mother now recalls the well to which the women of the village would daily carry their jugs to be filled. It was a "meeting place for the latest village news, sharing, and advice. As the water was a life-giving resource for the body, the woman's and her family's, so the sharing was a resource, a comfort, a renewal of a woman's spirit."

It is this women's well of shared experience that has come to be so important to me in my passage through menopause. For I have discovered it to be a fresh and deep source for life changes. My own thirst and personal desire to draw from that well has led me to experience there "the flow of Being"[3] that is the source of all Life. This book is an offering that comes out of my experience at that well. It is for anyone who seeks to understand this life passage and its potential for growth. It is my offering of encouragement to my sister pilgrims.

We each make our individual trip to the well, carrying our own jug, amphora, or bucket. Yet when we meet there, we discover that there is much that we share as we make this journey through menopause. It is my hope that you will discover the women's well and spend time there by yourself and with others.

> We come to the Well
> for refreshment
>
> Each one in turn
> lets the bucket down
> and draws deeply
>   from the Life-giving water.
>
> In this way we meet our sisters
> and together name
> that which is.
>
> So doing
> we strengthen one another
> to return home
> to share the water
>   the Life-giving water that we bear.

I. Discovering the Well of Our Experience

1. Trusting Our Experience

E very woman between forty and fifty-five has the opportunity to learn about herself in deep and life-changing ways. During that time most of us begin the process that leads to menopause. Our bodies begin to get our attention in new ways.

Those of us who have previously relied on a regular rhythm of menstrual cycles begin to experience irregularity. We become conscious of a need for regular mammograms. Gynecological check-ups often raise questions and suggest procedures that involve decisions about surgery and/or hormone treatment. Those of us who have had to deal with gynecological problems over the years, who may have had hysterectomies earlier, also experience physical changes. Our changing bodies remind us of our mortality.

In past generations the whole experience surrounding menopause was referred to as *the Change*. It was viewed, and therefore often lived out, as something to dread, fear, or, at the very least, endure. This negative experience was very private, rarely talked about except with one's male physician. Women today may have had a grandmother who went away to some hospital because she was "going through the Change." Our own mothers acknowledge a lonely span of years in which they did not feel like themselves. They did not like themselves, but somehow they made it through — alone, or with a doctor's hand-holding, or perhaps tranquilizing. My mother had to have a hysterectomy. Many women at that time were told that it was medically necessary. As one woman reported after she had asked her mother about her hysterectomy and menopause: "She doesn't remember anything. She just got rid of her uterus, and so did all my aunts, I think, but they never talked to each other about it."

As recently as the 1960s, this negative constellation of thoughts and experience was underscored by male doctors who described menopause as the end of womanhood and femininity. The "hope of feminine fulfillment" lay in estrogen treatment, which was the answer to keeping women "feminine forever."[1] No wonder women feared aging!

At the same time young women in the '60s, who had experienced natural childbirth, were discovering that they knew a lot about how to cooperate with the natural processes of their bodies. They began to trust their own experience. These same women, now in their forties and fifties, are bringing that experience to menopause and writing books about it. They are medical doctors, psychologists, psychotherapists, nutritionists, political activists, poets, and seekers who are encouraging women to grow with their changing bodies. They are challenging us to make responsible decisions regarding our own health care and to share our experiences with one another.

Not long ago many of us believed that doctors would guide us through whatever health problems we might have. They were the ultimate resources. This mystique was encouraged by many people in our lives. Recently a friend of mine at the age of forty-five was going to have a major operation. Her eighty-year-old father reminded her to "be sure and do what the doctor says." Even though we may not be told this explicitly, there is often a childhood memory something like mine: "Well, we'd better call the Doctor," said my mother, as she put her hand on my forehead or read the thermometer. I thought to myself, "Whew! He'll make me feel better." I was lucky enough to have him come to my bedside. I remember waiting to hear our doorbell. Then I would hear Doctor Robinson's footsteps on the front stairs. Finally he would come into my room and sit right beside me on the bed. His magic black bag made a special sound when he opened it. As he reached in to get his cold stethescope, a smell was released that told me once again: *You are going to get better.* Many of us still long for this kind of reassurance.

A woman who is involved in the medical field as a physical therapist recently learned of the death of her "esteemed Boston gynecologist." He had seen her through some very difficult times. She described his death as leaving "a large void in my medical care as I approached the menopause years." In her search to find a new doctor who "communicated well and one who seemed competent," she began to realize that even well-known doctors in the field often assume that women want their physicians to take over and manage their cases. "Many times physicians think we want a cure, when actually what we want is an understanding of *why* our bodies are doing whatever they are doing," she noted. One doctor, a physician at a teaching hospital, saw her for five minutes after an exam. She asked him to tell her what to expect about menopause: "He simply said, *Menopause is when you stop having menstruation.* Period. This physician is extremely well known in the medical world of Boston!" she said. We want to be respected and listened to by a health care professional. We want information well beyond the simple explanation: Menopause is when you stop menstruating. We want to know: What's happening in my body?

Doctors and health care professionals give a wide range of responses when asked this question. Their answers come out of their own orientation and particular point of view regarding health care. One end of the spectrum was reported to me by a friend whose doctor declared: "Menopause is a disease. It is not natural." As such he treats this "disease" in the same way he would diabetes or low thyroidism or any other endocrine deficiency disease. The other end of the spectrum was presented in one of the first books that I found dealing with the subject, Jane Fonda's *Women Coming of Age*. In this popular manual, Fonda explains that around menopause the "reproductive endocrine network" is moving through a time of "disequilibrium and readjustment." She presents it as a natural process of realignment.[2]

This made sense to me. I had been searching books for words that would reflect the sense that I held in my body. I was experiencing changes that were upsetting because I was not prepared for them. I did not understand them, but they did feel natural. Having studied child development, I was familiar with the idea of disequilibrium preceding change and growth into a new stage of equilibrium. I could apply it to my approaching menopause.

Given the range of viewpoints, we do need to have information that we can process on our own. Reading several books will give an idea of the various viewpoints. We then need to make sense out of this information in relation to our own experience. It is important to be aware of the bias of whatever is being presented. Media reporting in particular often presents only one side of an issue and data that supports one perspective. Winnifred Cutler and her associates underscore the importance of trusting our own experience in their book written from a biomedical point of view: *Menopause: A Guide for Women and the Men Who Love Them.*

> Once you are alert to the biases, you should develop a health maintenance plan that will most effectively serve your needs through your menopause. To do this requires that you get in tune with your body. . . .
>
> You will need the strength of will to secure the type of health care which you decide is best for *you*. . . . To maximize your health, you must take responsibility for yourself because only *you* can know how good you feel.[3]

In the process of developing our own "health maintenance plan," finding a doctor with whom we can work is very important. Sadja Greenwood, author of *Menopause Naturally*, reminds her readers that the word *doctor* comes from the Latin word for "teacher."

Her approach is an encouragement to seek out a doctor who would be open to a teacher-learner relationship that involves cooperative sharing of information and mutual respect.

One woman took three years to find a person with whom she could work in this way. Along the way she gathered information and experience, both positive and negative. "I realized that I had begun to take things into my own hands. I had to find a person and a place that I was comfortable with for the long haul." The word "manager" comes from the root word *manus*, which means "hand." When we begin to take things into our own hands, we become managers of our own health maintenance.

It does take strength of will to persevere in the process of securing the kind of health care that seems best for us. Each person's experience is very individual. For some women there may be minimal changes as they move through menopause. They may be able to work along with their regular family doctor or the person who delivered their babies, feeling that their questions and concerns are met with respect. Whatever our situation, there is some real satisfaction in taking on the role of manager of our own health maintenance plan. Once we accept this and are willing to put our energy into it, we become aware again that we have options and choices. This awareness is empowering. One woman told me,

> I had been experiencing irregular periods for a while. I went to our family doctor and asked him about these signs. My question was, Is this the time of my life or is something seriously wrong? He told me that the definite way of knowing that I was going through menopause was through a blood test, which he took. He then said that perhaps this was the time to discuss hormone replacement therapy. "What do you think?" he asked. Given my history of cystic breasts and varicose veins, I replied, "I'm not a candidate." He said, "All right," that those were contraindications, but he was concerned that I might need H.R.T. later on, as osteoporosis runs in my family. He stressed the importance of movement and exercise as helps to strengthen bones.

In stating "I'm not a candidate," this woman was taking seriously her own health management. She had done a lot of reading, had gathered information from others, and had found a doctor who respected her opinion. He recognized her as the one who knew her body, the one who would make the necessary related decisions. However, what is most important is that she *trusted her own experience.* She said, "I am not taking anything for now. As things progress, I shall update my choices. I am confident in my advisors and my knowledge."

We have the opportunity at this time in our lives to develop confidence in ourselves as our own health managers. Talking with other women about books and articles that we have read, about doctors and other health care professionals, helps to add to the resource pool of information. Some women choose to do this by joining a menopause support group. Others initiate this kind of information gathering with their friends. This is also a good time to talk with older women, asking them about their experience. It gives a perspective to our own experience and that of our peers. It is a time to draw on the shared experience of the women's community.

In the past decade many good books and articles on menopause have been written by women as part of that shared experience. The reading list at the end of this chapter names and briefly describes some of the resources currently available. I have found many of them helpful in my search for answers to my questions.

I discovered, for instance, that what was feeling like a long process of continual change is clinically called "the female climacteric," which refers to a continuum of change that surrounds the actual ceasing of menstruation. It has three recognized phases: *Perimenopause*, which is the time in which our bodies are preparing for menopause. Our ovaries are producing fewer and fewer eggs. Hormones work overtime to compensate, which can cause various bodily changes in menstrual and related conditions. *Menopause* proper is the actual ceasing of our menses, which is determined when we have no menstrual bleeding for one year. *Postmenopause* refers to the time following the end of our menstruation when our bodies are readjusting to the changes in our hormonal system. The length of time for this whole process of rebalancing varies greatly as do the physical signs of these changes.

I have also discovered how important it is to develop my own philosophical approach to the time surrounding menopause. A teacher of adolescents made a similar discovery. She was having difficulty with hot flashes, especially during school. She told a group of women about how she tried to hide the dripping sweat that came unbidden during the day. After talking and laughing together about this common experience, she went back to her school, deciding to acknowledge to her class what was happening to her. Doing this, she soon noticed that her hot flashes lessened in intensity. She later commented to the group on this shift in herself: "It seems a dramatic confirmation of the truth that what you resist, you get more of, and when you accept a situation, then you can go about freeing yourself."

It seems true for me and the women with whom I have shared this experience that what we hold, believe, and envision about this time in our lives can be as important as the answers that we find. Reading several different resources can be very helpful as we seek answers to our specific questions regarding our own bodily changes.

Resources for Menopause

Cameron, Anne. *Daughters of Copper Woman*. Vancouver, British Columbia: Press Gang Publishers, 1981.

Members of a society of women that began before recorded history share for the first time stories that have been passed down through generations of Nootka women on Vancouver Island. The author's poetic sense conveys a reverence for the natural rhythms of women's bodies, the shared experience of honoring those rhythms, and a true enjoyment of womanhood.

Cobb, Janine O'Leary. *Understanding Menopause*. Toronto: Key Porter Books Limited, 1989.

One of the best all-around resources available. As Cobb says in her introduction, "Understanding what is happening will, I think, allow you to re-establish cordial relations with a body and mind that may be temporarily out of whack, enabling you to manage your menopause with confidence."

Cutler, Winnifred B. *Hysterectomy—Before and After*. New York: HarperCollins, 1990.

A comprehensive guide to preventing, preparing for, and maximizing health after a hysterectomy.

Cutler, Winnifred Berg, Celso-Ramon Garcia, and David A. Edwards. *Menopause: A Guide for Women and the Men Who Love Them*. New York: W. W. Norton & Co., 1983, 1985, 1991.

Hormone replacement therapy is presented as having some real benefits "when experienced with full knowledge and attendence to various dangers." The book encourages women to develop a health maintenance plan that serves their needs through menopause.

Doress, Paula Brown, Diana Laskin Siegal, and the Midlife and Older Womens' Book Project. *Ourselves Growing Older: Women Aging with Knowledge and Power*. New York: Simon & Schuster, 1987.

With an emphasis on the positive potential of the second half of life, the book is a resource on many subjects and concerns that face women. The chapter on menopause is a good place to begin. Related subjects are covered in greater detail in separate chapters.

Downing, Christine. *Journey Through Menopause: A Personal Rite of Passage*. New York: Crossroad, 1987.

An account of Downing's personal saga that encourages other women to experience the life passage of menopause as a spiritual journey that is both a body event and a "soul event, which means letting it be transformative."

Fonda, Jane. *Women Coming of Age*. New York: Simon & Schuster, 1984.

A program of well-being for middle-aged women, presenting the hormonal system during the years surrounding menopause as "realigning itself . . . into a new stage of balance." Specific nutritional and physical exercise suggestions are helpful contributions.

Greenwood, Sadja. *Menopause, Naturally: Preparing for the Second Half of Life*. San Francisco: Volcano Press, 1989.

The author is associated with women's health programs professionally. Her knowledge as a general practitioner draws on interest in both Eastern and Western medicine. She has personally explored nutrition and exercise in her own passage through menopause. Sound and balanced information is presented in an enjoyable way.

Lark, Susan M. *Women's Menopause Self-Help Book*. Berkeley: Celestial Arts, 1990.

This "Woman's Guide to Feeling Wonderful" looks at "all natural" treatments for symptoms of menopause: diet, vitamins, herbs, stress reduction, exercise, accupressure, massage, yoga, neurovascular and neurolymphatic holding points, and estrogen replacement therapy. An encouragement to put together your own program.

Nachtigall, Lila, and Joan Rattner Heilman. *Estrogen: The Facts Can Change Your Life*. New York: Harper & Row, 1986, 1991.

A physician who specializes in reproductive endocrinology presents the case for estrogen replacement therapy as "safe when used correctly — in low doses, combined with progesterone, individualized for each woman, monitored regularly through gynecological examinations." "It is dangerous to start E.R.T. in perimenopause," Nachtigal warns, though it is recognized as helpful for many of the conditions experienced by women in menopause.

Reitz, Rosetta. *Menopause: A Positive Approach.* New York: Penguin Books, 1979.
Women ranging in age from twenty-five to ninety-five speak about "sex and aging, lovemaking, hormones, nutrition, and more." Their experience before and after menopause was gathered from interviews and menopause workshops. Much information is still very relevant as is the positive approach. It is dated regarding hormone replacement therapy.

Sumrall, Amber Coverdale, and Dena Taylor, editors. *Women of the 14th Moon: Writings on Menopause.* Freedom, California: Crossing Press, 1991.
A "collection of inspiring, painful, funny, informative, and poetic first-person accounts of menopause" gathered by the editors to encourage other women to claim "this part of their life as vital and empowering."

Trien, Susan Flamholtz. *Change of Life: The Menopause Handbook.* New York: Fawcett-Columbine, Ballentine Books, 1986.
A health writer provides a handbook with helpful charts and diagrams addressing medical topics, emotional and life issues, and "well-care" advice. A good resource with an excellent bibliography.

Utian, Wolf H., and Ruth S. Jacobowitz. *Managing Your Menopause.* New York: Prentice Hall, 1990.
The importance of a woman's weighing the risks and the benefits of hormone replacement therapy is presented in a helpful way as part of this doctor's program for individually designed health-care maintenance. The Utian Menopause Management program developed out of twenty years of experience working with women.

Wolfe, Honora Lee. *Second Spring: A Guide to Healthy Menopause Through Traditional Chinese Medicine.* Boulder, Colorado: Blue Poppy Press, 1990.
A book written for laywomen, presenting traditional Chinese medicine's understanding of menopause. The theory, explanations, self-help measures, and various therapies offer an alternative to the Western medical approach.

Newsletters

A Friend Indeed for women in the prime of life.
Edited by Janine O'Leary Cobb, this monthly comes with topical information related specifically to menopause; reviews of up-to-date research findings and/or publications that can help women "to make knowledgeable decisions." Back issues are indexed and available for specific concerns. Write *A Friend Indeed* Publications, Inc., Box 515, Place du Parc Station, Montreal, Quebec H2W 2P1, Canada. For a free introductory issue, send a self-addressed stamped envelop to Box 1710, Champlain, New York 12919-1710.

Hot Flash is the official newsletter of the National Action Forum for Mid-life and Older Women.
Relevant concerns including signs of menopause are presented in four volumes a year. Write *Hot Flash*, Newsletter for Older Women, c/o Dr. Jane Porchino, Box 816, Stony Brook, New York 11790-0609.

2. Sharing Our Experience

As women, our experience starts with our bodies, and it is there that our knowing differs from the experience of men. We become women with a bodily change. We know what it is to be a woman through our bodies.

Tribal rites of initiation for girls begin with the first menstruation. Because of the bodily changes, the young woman's transformation needs less ceremonial markings than a young man's. Boys' assumption of adulthood is not a bodily experience; therefore it needs social and conventional delineation.[1] A girl, however, becomes a woman through bodily knowing. She is the first to know. It is her experience.

It is also our everyday experience that our bodies are a source of deep inner knowing. Until recently we have not been encouraged to speak from this knowledge and, thus, have not trusted our own experience or acted out of it. One reason that we distrusted ourselves is that our culture conveyed a message that the experience of menstrual bleeding was bad, negative, "the curse." A negative interpretation was placed on the Jewish practice of a woman ritually cleansing herself during and after her time of menstruation. When the Hebrew Scriptures refer to the practice of women separating from the community during menstruation, the words are usually translated to say that it is because the women are "unclean."

The Christian tradition took this further and understood menstruation as being "dirty" and a sign of sinfulness.[2] This antisexual teaching rooted in Western culture has been a source of feelings of isolation and shame among women. This separation of body and spirit has also been a loss for our whole culture and perhaps for our planet. It is, therefore, exciting to be living in a time when new voices are being heard, voices of women encouraging other women to trust, speak, and act from our own experience.

Voices from other cultures, indigenous women's societies, have much to say to us about the sacredness of our bodies' experiences. On Vancouver Island the Nootka women were taught to grow with their bodies by following their bodies' natural rhythms, gaining wisdom from that source. For them, as recorded by Anne Cameron, menstruation was a holy and sacred time, a time for prayer and contemplation. It was a time in the natural rhythm of life when women went to the waiting house to be joined by others who were also menstruating.[3]

In the Laguna Pueblo Native American tradition, blood was sacred, "the water of life," evidence of women's life-giving power. It was taboo for men to be near women at this time, as well as during labor, because "what is empowered [the blood] in a ritual sense is not to be touched or approached by any who are weaker than the power itself, lest they suffer negative consequences from contact. . . . so women were held in awe and respect."[4]

This sense of awe is being recovered by women who are beginning to share their experience with each other. Not only is the sacred quality of our natural body rhythms being respected, but also we are discovering the powerful experience of sharing this with other women of all ages. There is a longing for the waiting house or "moon hut" experience, as it is called in some cultures. I have experienced this longing in gatherings of women, when one woman begins talking to another about her experience around menopause. Within minutes others who are tuned into their own experience pick up the waves and are drawn to the conversation. The energy level goes up as several women begin to speak freely of what they know. Unlike our mothers' generation, we are now giving ourselves permission to talk openly, to share experience, and to listen to each other.

I remember well the first workshop that I led exploring "Menopause as an Opportunity." The agenda was to discuss the physical and emotional changes that we were having and to open to the deeper movement of letting go into something new. We talked about the signs (often called "symptoms") that we were experiencing, the myths of menopause with which many of us grew up, and the facts that are now available through the increasing number of good books, journals, and newsletters.

The room filled with laughter, empathy, outbursts of anger, and moments of tears — so much energy that at one point I opened the door. The space was not big enough to contain the experience that we shared. This group decided to continue meeting on a regular basis to learn more about this life passage. We had discovered in that first day how important it is to share our experience and to encourage others to do the same. In doing this we were recognizing the significance of each other's experience.

Many women who have grown up in the Judeo-Christian tradition are reclaiming a sense of what Matthew Fox has named "original blessing."[5] For some of us, discovering the sacredness of our own bodies has been a painful process of emerging from restrictive doctrines set forth by male authorities — religious and otherwise. A woman who had worked very hard to understand and experience liberation from that kind of restriction was part of a group that was developing the theme of the body as sacred. I vividly remember her igniting energy as she exclaimed, "My God, my body is a sacred place. I love my body!" A contagious fire of celebration passed around the circle, a shared sense of life-giving energy. We recognized the significance of this experience of great joy for her.

When we share these moments of awakening with one another, we take risks. I felt this myself as I shared an experience with a friend. I had been going through a period of intense self-doubt and anxiety. As I often do when I feel that I am not enough for a task, I had pushed myself all the harder. I became aware of the toll that my body had taken under the pushing, driving force of my fearfulness.

Early one morning I felt a deep need to be compassionate toward my body, which had carried me through the storm of my fears. I felt moved to really look at my body, to see my body, to see myself just as I am. I felt a longing to express my love and caring for my body.

Bringing a mirror into my workroom, I began to look at myself. I looked at my body from top to toe, exploring myself with great reverence. Time stood still. I looked at myself for a long time in the mirror. Slowly I began to dress myself. As I put my socks over my toes, which I touched one by one and marveled at their construction, I felt like I was dressing a very small infant, marveling at her body, as I put each piece of clothing on. I kept looking at my face with its wrinkles, life lines, scars, my face loving my body, my face holding me in such tender regard.

This was a holy moment for me in which I knew the presence of the Divine, embodied in the temple of my being. For a long time I kept this experience to myself, unsure that its deep significance to me would be understood. When I ventured to share my sense of meeting the Divine in this bodily way, I experienced the gift of being heard and understood by my friend.

One of the most important things that we can do for each other at this time of life is to listen for and recognize the significance of each other's experience, for our experiences will vary. The ways in which we encounter the sacred may be quite different. Whether as friends, pilgrims along the way, or members of a menopause support group, we can encourage one another to trust and claim our experience as significant.

The changes going on in our bodies evoke all kinds of feelings. At a time of unpredictable periods and very heavy bleeding near the beginning of perimenopause, I remember deep feelings of sadness. I wrote them in my journal:

tears tears flowing
    as my life blood goes
        a continuous outpouring

clots of blood
    large and dark
        slipping from my womb
           which once bore
                such
                vibrancy!

The process of letting go of the childbearing years for some women can involve all the stages of grief, as Elisabeth Kubler-Ross has outlined them.[6] One woman who has loved being a wife and mother stopped menstruating quite suddenly at forty. She kept "putting a pad on each month." It was too soon for her. She had not had time to prepare herself. She held on. She did not want what was so to be. This kind of denial is often followed by the other stages of grief: anger, bargaining, depression, and finally acceptance.

Women who have not borne children by choice or by circumstance also experience grief at this time of bodily awareness. A woman who is a member of a religious order spoke of the period of time in which she anticipated a possible hysterectomy. She knew that it was a time of "mourning and anticipatory grief . . . over the thought that my fertile time of life was coming to a close." Another woman who came to a conscious choice not to have a child spoke of the hurt that accompanied that decision: "When I would see a pregnant woman, I would be jealous, and I hurt inside. The hurt was for the intimacy that could bring forth a child." This was an acknowledged loss for her.

"I always thought that I would have a child," said a woman who is in her mid-forties. Recently she experienced a shift inside herself to not wanting a child. As she reflected on this, she realized that the healing work that she had been doing with her own inner child had helped to create this change. "This work has helped me to know that my loss in not bearing children has not been total, for I have developed creatively anyway." Her experience of this inner shift felt "like a release of energy . . . like a freedom." All the energy that had been tied up in "the hormonal urge or primordial passion" to give birth to a child has been released. "Now I know I don't have to do that," she said. "Always before it was like maintaining an extra room in my house, a baby room, anticipating a child to come. It took energy for that, and now it is available for other things."

For others, the loss is not so much in relation to never bearing children, but it comes as they anticipate the end of menstruation, which has been a profound experience for them. This was true for a woman who said, "I have my period to be a whole person, to be connected to the earth and part of the cycle of life." Or as her friend put it, "Ever since I was eighteen or nineteen, I have enjoyed the feelings in my womb. I just knew there was something special about it. I could feel the sacredness."

I am sure that some of my grief had to do with fearing that this bodily way of connecting with the sacred would also cease with the ending of my menses. My body had taught me about letting go and flowing with the rhythms of the universe. It had offered me an experience of knowing what it is to trust and release my attempts at control. I have known in a physical-sensing-earthy-bloodflow-and-aching way my oneness with all creation and the Creator.

This sense of bodily connection with the sacred or the Divine was put into words by a woman who said, "My period has been my intimate connection with Mystery. My period always felt good to me like a cleansing, a sacrifice, a shedding for new honoring, my body doing what it needs to do. . . . I love the homeliness of it." The process of grieving the cessation of our menses when the experience of menstruation has had this sacred quality is very important. As one of these women said, "It's like approaching a new mystery . . . like life after death."

At this time in life, for those who do not have children there can be a sense of loss in knowing there will not be grandchildren. "The reality is there on holidays — you don't have the family connection," said one woman. Another woman shared her sadness in not having children to whom she could pass things on. She spoke of "the on-goingness of ourselves: What I have brought into life, things about myself that I treasure, things I've made, like a poem, or things that I've learned. Maybe that is narcissistic, but I don't think so. I think it is self-valuing." Another woman acknowledged this loss and added her thoughts: "My closest connections are not family connections. We have to learn to make connections in another way. We just have to do sooner what all women do. We really need to choose our own parents, brothers and sisters, and children."

Allowing ourselves to feel the feelings of loss and sadness enables us to move toward letting go and the acceptance of what is so. There is much involved in that movement from denial to letting go and acceptance. Letting go is a bodily lesson that the womb has been teaching us since we became young women. Each month we have been reminded that we are not in control, that we are part of a rhythm that goes beyond us and connects us with the moon rhythms of the universe. The changes that we experience, that are related to the hormonal rebalancing process, also challenge our sense of control. This is particularly true for those of us who have known good health and felt in charge of ourselves in that domain. As with pregnancy, our womb at this time in our lives can be a place where we encounter the Divine in our experience. We are reminded by our wombs' changes that ultimately we are not in control, but rather we are cooperators with the Creator in the process of creation.

Many of us experience and meet the Divine through our womb's dis-ease, or potential disease. The first time that lumps were discovered in my breasts, I was aware of a heightened sense of the preciousness of life, experiencing it as truly a gift. The experiences of having gynecological checkups that raise questions and propose solutions having to do with our breasts or things like a D&C, hormone replacement therapy, a hysterectomy, and/or treatment for uterine cancer force us to face our mortality. There is grief in that, and it is often experienced in all of its stages. Any woman who has dealt with these concerns can recall becoming enraged at a medical secretary, lab technician, doctor, friend, relative, or perfect stranger, and after the fact realizing that the intensity of anger was not proportionate to the situation. The outburst may have been carrying the heavy freight of looking at death perhaps for the first time. Our wombs often give us the opportunity to walk with our fears through "the valley of the shadow of death" (Psalm 23:4) and to encounter more deeply than ever before the sacredness of life.

During the passage through menopause, when women can choose to become one with their bodies, some women find that this choice opens memories of physical and/or sexual abuse. The grief involved in this remembering needs tender healing support and therapy. *Therapaeia*, Christine Downing points out, is the Greek root word meaning attention of the kind one gives to the sacred.[7]

There is also a darkness for some women at this time that has been called depression and is often treated as such medically. Sometimes that is appropriate. One woman who was never able to have children because of a physical condition became very depressed as she neared her fiftieth year. She was given medication by her doctor to ease the symptoms of her depression, but she had never directly expressed with friends and family her anger and deep sadness over the loss of the opportunity to be a mother.

The recent work of developmental psychologists Irene Stiver and Jean Baker Miller sheds light on many women's experience. In a paper titled "From Depression to Sadness in Women's Psychotherapy," they make a clear and important distinction between sadness and depression. Sadness is a "feeling state," and depression is a "state in which feelings are hidden . . . a 'non-feeling state.'" They make the important point that often there is not a context in which feelings of sadness and loss can be expressed, in which the significance of that loss can be understood by those around us: "Sometimes the woman initially may have a sense of her feelings, but the people around her are conveying the strong message that she shouldn't have them. There's no reason to have them; so if anything is wrong, it must be that something is wrong with her."[8]

Our mothers may have experienced this kind of emotional atmosphere when they went through their menopause. Given the lack of empathy or validation of their experience of loss, it is no wonder that many women reacted in a stoic fashion. Others who could not manage that facade appeared to be depressed or erratic in their behavior and sometimes were considered to be going crazy. We now have the opportunity to be in a context where feelings are acceptable and where empathy for the significance of our losses is present.

Our feelings of loss will vary. Some of us may grieve the loss of our role as childbearers and mothers; others may connect with what it has meant to not have children. Some of us may grieve the loss of a sense of control over our bodies that have always supported our desired level of activity. Others may be discovering the sacredness of our bodies in a new way, connecting with past pain over the loss of our sense of original blessing. But when we enter a context where the significance of our loss is received, be it in a friendship, a group, or a therapy session, we feel less isolated. Then we feel more active, less self-blaming, more energized and expressive. Having that kind of experience, we can then find ways to express ourselves to those with whom we share our lives. For they, too, need to recognize the significance of our loss. Enabling them to feel connected is part of the gift that we have to offer. The men in our lives and younger women, friends, and health professionals need to hear from us. But first we need to hear ourselves.

3. Renaming Our Experience

Many women are now realizing that the span of time surrounding menopause is much more than a medically defined continuum of change within a woman's reproductive system. We are discovering together that, for us, it is a life passage that needs to be recognized as such and honored by moving it from a passive state to an active state.

"The Change" was used by our mothers' generation as a noun for something that, like the plague and the curse, happened *to* a person. According to *Webster's New Collegiate Dictionary*, the verb "to change" comes from a Celtic root word meaning "to exchange, to give up something for something else." That process of letting go so that something new can come forth is a deeply spiritual movement. We as women have the opportunity to know that movement in a bodily way through our own experience, which is not passive but rather creative. As we choose actively to engage in changing, we experience a transformation of life energy.

We can rename our experience, choosing to discover our bodies as life-giving and thus sacred, connecting us with the Divine. Many of us now in mid-life were not aware of this potential for spiritual learning that our bodies offered to us in our early years when we began our menses. We had no waiting house in which to receive this knowledge. Few of us at ten, twelve, or thirteen, on our own, would have recognized the spiritual movement of being acted upon by nature, becoming one with nature, as we let go into the rhythms of shedding and replenishing. Nor would we have been aware of nature's amazing balancing process. "It takes about seven years from the first menstrual period until a woman is fully fertile, and it takes about seven years for the reverse process (total infertility) to be complete."[1] The number seven has long been a symbol of creative fullness. That fullness is experienced when we choose to be conscious and become one with our bodies.

The seven-year span ending our fertility gives us a real opportunity. During this time we can learn more fully to trust our bodies, to re-member the whole of our experience through our bodies, and to learn from them. As we do this, we can choose to cooperate with our bodies' processes, thus holding our bodies sacred. Engaging in this way with our passage through menopause, we can participate in re-naming. We can create new names for our own experience.

This was Christine Downing's intention as she went on her *Journey Through Menopause*, which resulted in the book of that title:

> I don't want to get around it. I want to live it. I don't want to "treat" it or "cure" it, though I do want to honor it with curiosity, and with "therapy" (*therapaeia*), attention of the kind one devotes to sacred mysteries. I want to allow menopause to be a soul event, which means letting it be transformative.[2]

In her preparatory research, she read both male and female medical and psychological accounts of the climacteric period, written from the perspective of medical pathology, seeing menopause as a deficiency disease. This view is based on the assumptions that femininity equals motherhood, that menstruation and menopause refer only to reproductive processes, and that the womb is solely an organ for making babies. Many of us have been affected by this focus. The extreme sense of loss and ending that some women feel as they approach menopause is closely related to this medical view.

The narrow interpretation of femininity that has dominated our culture has not only been hurtful to individual women, but it has limited all of us in our understanding of womanhood. It has been exciting to meet with groups of women who are uncovering these one-dimensional views and challenging them with the evidence of their own lives. One woman who, through various life choices, does not have children said with great clarity and conviction, "The view of our womb as solely a place of reproduction is a limited and limiting view. It's a small man's small idea! It's coming from a sense of deficiency." She was joined by another woman who also chose not to have children:

> It is an over-simplification of the womb to see it as reproductive. It is so focused and logical and male. Women's knowing is womblike. Women know our womb has multiple functions. Childbearing is only one aspect of its functions. That's why making love during menstruation is so marvelous. It's when you are not able to make babies and when what you are doing is making love.

A married woman who had wanted very much to have children and was unable to do so recognized her own feelings and reactions to the limited cultural understanding of womanhood as she approached menopause: "I feel relief. At last my friends will be learning what I have been coming to accept during the time that they were bearing and raising children and becoming grandmothers." Women who have not borne children know the broader meaning of being a woman that others of us will come to know in our passage through menopause. Women who have chosen lifestyles other than marriage, and those whose experience of womanhood has not involved childbearing, have much to share with those for whom children have been a major focus.

Our Native American sisters have always celebrated the experience of woman that goes beyond procreation. The Spirit that pervades all creation, as they believe, has many names, but "at the center of all is Woman, and no thing is sacred (cooked, ripe as the Keres Indians of Laguna Pueblo say it) without her blessing, her thinking."[3] Far beyond a fertility goddess, she is the Supreme Spirit, a "true creatrix for she is thought itself, from which all else is born." A Keres ceremonial prayer recorded by Paula Gunn Allen in *The Sacred Hoop* speaks of "Woman" as "mother of us all, after Her, mother earth follows, in fertility, in holding, and in taking again us back to her breast."[4] Allen speaks for her people who see the power of woman as the center of the universe that "is both heart (womb) and thought (creativity)."[5]

This expansive sense of womanhood encourages a much broader understanding of woman as mother. Reflecting on the relationship between our womb and our creativity, some artists agreed: "While some women were learning to be mothers, we were learning to be artists. Being a mother is like being an artist. We both learn to value life by giving attention." Another artist whose life choices have not led her to bearing children added her insight:

> We are mothers! I feel connected to all children — as well as the children that I know. I feel close to them. Motherhood is not just biological. It is a gift! We do a kind of mothering as well as our own creation. It's like being a special edition for children instead of a daily newspaper.

One woman named her experience of her womb's cycle and renamed the womb as the source of creativity:

> All women have the same process. It just doesn't look the same. It is not re-production that we are talking about, whether it's babies or anything else. It's not producing

something over and over again. . . . It's creation. Our cycle is a creative process. It includes elation, expansion, creation, and then you are immensely depressed when you are separated from that which you have made. You ask yourself: Will I be fertile again? Our womb is where creativity comes!

Jean Shinoda Bolen, author of *Goddesses in Everywoman*, suggests a mythic way of viewing our wombs and the transformation in our bodies. She sees the process as a pilgrimage, the purpose of which is to "quicken the Divine" in the pilgrim. She suggests that woman's spiritual pilgrimage is an inward one led by a new symbol for the Holy Grail, the womb. Like the chalice, it holds life-giving blood that is sacred.[6] The object of the quest becomes no longer something out there, sought after in the fashion of the medieval knights on pilgrimage. We ourselves bear the chalice within. Journeying to our own experience within our bodies, we can meet the Divine.

One woman named her experience in this way: "My womb is not a metaphor for creation. It is not a symbol or an image. This physical being, my womb, *is* creation and connects me with the Goddess." For each of us, the naming will be our own.

Dreams can get our attention and help us in this naming process as they speak to us from our unconscious, our deeper self. Sometimes dreams can be humorous, containing puns as a way of presenting information to our rational self. Other times they guide us to owning, claiming, and naming what is of real value in our lives.

Five years before I actually stopped menstruating, I had a dream that alerted me to the importance of claiming and naming my experience as I moved through the passage of menopause.

I have been in a car and realize that I need to get my things out of the car. I have a sense of urgency about that. I go to the car. It is parked on the brink of a hill overlooking the ocean. I am reaching in, getting bags, etc. I realize that my purse is on the dashboard. I reach in to get it, to retrieve it. The car starts moving forward. I grope around and find the brake just in time before the car goes over the hill.

I felt great relief on waking. I had a sense that the dream's message was this: If I do not retrieve what I most value, I may lose it "over the hill." For me it became very important to reclaim (or retrieve) my womb, which, like a purse, held great value for me, even during a time that has been referred to as "over the hill." This dream marked the beginning of my willingness to open to the Divine through my womb's experience.

Recognizing menopause as a "soul event" as well as a body event creates a more inclusive way of journeying through this passage. As we open ourselves to the changes taking place in our wombs, as we reflect, remember, grieve, rejoice, and live the changes, we engage the Divine. We become one with the Mystery of life itself when we become one with our own experience.

II. Drawing from the Women's Well

way. . . . I have a strange feeling you heard me before I started. You heard me to my own story."[3] We can do this for each other by listening with reverence; we can do this for ourselves by remembering.

Remembering our experience before menstruation is important for women approaching menopause. Menarche, the onset of menstruation, and menopause, the actual cessation of the menses, are two balancing movements in our bodies' natural rhythms. There is a deep connection between the times of beginning and ending our physical fertility. I have discovered for myself and from others that there is much to learn and to gain from re-membering our experience as young girls.

One woman connected with the importance of her menses to her as a girl in her late teens:

> When I was sixteen and still didn't have my period, my mother and I went to a doctor who told me that I probably would never get my period, or if I did get it, I probably wouldn't be able to get pregnant. My mother didn't respond at all. She didn't like her period and called it "the curse." So I was scared of having children, replicating my mother's experience and my terrible childhood.
>
> But when I was nineteen, I did get my period, and I felt terrific. I had a sense that I was intimately connected to a process that nobody — not me, not my mother, a man, society — can control. It had to do with rhythm and it was organic. . . . It was *my* menstruation.

Many of us have negative memories about our preparation for menstruation, and some of us feel sadness about what we gave up as childhood seemed to end. Our experience, negative or positive, is part of our story. It is what was so. Sharing these experiences with other women offers opportunity to include and not forget. Accepting what was so and learning from that experience, we actually become freer to make choices about this time of life as we approach our menopause. As a woman in her late forties remembered, "My mother's message was: Being a woman is becoming like me. So I became my mother. It was her menses, not mine. Maybe that is why I want to really experience myself in this passage."

The lack of positive preparation for the experience of menstruation left some of us as young girls feeling a sense of shame. A woman in one group recalled how "scared" she was as she began to bleed:

> For several days I stained my underpants and tried to hide the bleeding. I didn't tell anyone. One day at school, over the loudspeaker, I was called to the nurse's office. My mother was there. She had found my underwear in the laundry. I felt ashamed. When I returned to the room, I felt embarrassed. I realize now that she wanted to protect me from that very thing, but she was operating out of her own fear.

Many of our mothers were not in touch with their own bodies. Their attempts to help us often carried fears and negative feelings about being a woman. This was the experience of one woman now in her late fifties: "This is what my mother said: *Here's a pad and don't get pregnant!* That was it."

The absence of personal sharing among women was the result of the uneasiness of so many adult women in our mothers' generation. Bodies, bodily functions, and anything sexual was most often very private. Even female health professionals conveyed information without their own involvement. Remembering this, another group member shared her experience of one such impersonal presentation:

> We were shown a movie in school and given a little booklet that the fifth-grade teacher told us that we should take right home and that he never wanted to see it in school again. The school nurse gave a talk and answered questions that anyone could put forth. No one really told me her experience, what happened, and how she felt. My mother's explanation was that menstruation was God's way of getting rid of extra blood in a woman's body, not anything that had to do with me as a person. As far as I knew God

was a superhuman man, and this was one more thing — right in the midst of me — that He was doing. I felt also that suddenly people knew something about me that I didn't know about myself, and there was a loss or taking away of privacy, autonomy. The actual first menstruation seemed to have absolutely nothing to do with what I had seen in the movie or been told. The blood was real, and there was feeling.

For many women there has been no women's well to come to, no place to learn in a personal way from the shared experience of others. There has been no "waiting house" or "moon hut" where older women who no longer bleed tend the younger women in their "moon time," while young girls assist, learning from these old wise women. Some women have been fortunate enough to have a positive beginning to menstruation as well, with mothers and older friends who celebrated that transition with them. Some women are creating their own rituals in honor of their daughters' first menstruation, marking it as a beginning of newness and possibility. And we now have the opportunity to journey through this ending in a different way that can be, and often is, a positive beginning.

Whatever our experience may have been in the months or years preceding menstruation, it has proven to be of great value for us in this life passage to remember and include now the young girl part of ourselves. Instead of leaving her experience behind, dropping it off, or *dis*-membering it, we need to include her in the way of the storyteller. We need to *re*-member for the purpose of preserving our wholeness. Inclusion of all the parts of our selves is a way of honoring our whole self. This whole-making, holy process is a sacred one. The passage of menopause offers us an opportunity to do this.

As I reflected on my experience, I realized that as I approached my menses I must have made a decision more like the wagon leader than the storyteller, for I really left behind my young girl self. I must have thought it was the only way to move on to the new destination that lay ahead: being a teenage girl. In remembering I also realized that dropping off this deeply valued part of myself left an emptiness, and from that empty feeling I hurried away. By journeying back and re-membering, I have reconnected with that young girl part of me and am influenced by her presence with me now in my fifties. She brings me new energy.

As a young girl, my greatest thrill and source of pride was being catcher on the boys' schoolyard baseball team. I loved it. Jeans, sloppy shirt, pigtails, my hat, and my glove were the accessories of a satisfied nine-year-old girl. Who would want that world to change? I surely didn't. What energy, enthusiasm, vitality! Life was a constant ballgame, and I was "one of the boys."

Somewhere around age eleven, it did change. When my girl-friends were covering their chests in the locker room and their mothers were buying them bras, I must have made my decision. I no longer caught for the boys. I organized a girls' team and became a short stop. My decision that I was not a boy, and therefore was a girl, was soon confirmed when I "got my period."

I moved on to dress in feminine ways and learned how to compete "appropriately." I became an organizer and a leader. I worked very hard at always being surrounded by girlfriends. I would fight to walk in the front of the pack of girls as we went down the street, up the street, and to the girls' room together. I was loud, mouthy, and sometimes cruel. I can see the group moving down the street, all talking at once. I tried hard always to be in front to keep people's attention.

I remember one girl at the back of the pack, always working hard to keep up, her pace being slower. She never complained. One day she was in the girls' room in one of the stalls. Several girls were with me. I opened the door to her stall. With teasing words, I exposed her. There was laughter. I was big stuff. That picture stays with me.

I told this tale first in my journal, and as I reconnected with this picture of myself, I had strong feelings. It was wonderful to remember that nine-year-old tomboy me, but I also felt something like grief. Along with a fondness for that vivacious child, I felt sadness at the loss of the simple, straightforward tomboy life and a longing to reclaim the vitality, enthusiasm, and directness of that pigtailed time. Cutting my braids and wearing a bra seemed to rein in that energy, only to have it come out in less direct, self- conscious, and sometimes hurtful ways.

As I discovered, connecting with a part of ourselves does often touch off strong feelings. I loved the tomboy. I felt grief over the loss of her and real remorse about my self-conscious insecurity in the following years. In the process of remembering, we come to a choice. We can acknowledge and recognize the feelings and then choose to let them go. We can also choose to embrace the feelings and the experience, to allow them to be present in our lives now.

When we make the choice to re-member and to include the experience of the young girl self, we free the energy of that part of us to join us and to be available in a new way for the choices that we are making at this time in our lives. As I worked with my feelings of sadness, they moved from grief to a longing for the vitality that was such a part of my young girl self. I have slowly become aware that by re-membering her, I can include her life energy now. That possibility adds a new dimension to my life in my fifties. I can look forward to discovering how that will be expressed.

Re-membering is important for preserving our wholeness. The process of reuniting parts of ourselves actually frees energy that has often been taken up in resistance or conflict between these parts. New energy comes when the parts begin working together, creating a whole. The Old English root word *hal* means "whole" or "health"; a derivative is healing. Re-membering, moving toward wholeness, can be truly healing.

There are many helpful ways to recall and remember: journal writing, sharing in a support group or with a close friend, therapist, or spiritual guide. One technique for remembering, which can be done individually or with another, was developed by Eugene Gendlin. Called "Focusing," it is a "change process"[4] based on a belief in bodily knowing, a trust in the wisdom that is carried in our bodies. It offers a way of sensing and trusting our bodies' responses to our experiences.

This process, which has been called "the art of allowing,"[5] has been particularly helpful to one celibate religious woman as a way to re-member and truly heal. Two major things happened about the same time in this woman's mid-life. At forty-seven she had a total hysterectomy — and she was introduced to "Focusing." She wrote a description in her journal of the first time that she used the technique for herself, and she shared it with me. Awakening one morning, she decided to follow the bodily sensation that she was having. When she asked herself the initial "Focusing" question: "Is there anything coming between me and feeling good right now?" she noticed her body's response: "A tightening in my incision."

> I put my hand on it and it was smooth — healing well. I checked in with my body again and explored what it was like inside. A question came, "Will I find emptiness, pain, and grief because those parts of me have been taken away?" No, I discovered something else to my surprise. Something seemed to say, "Remember me? I am that fear in you that you had in your teens — your fear of having children. Remember how your mother would get pregnant and be so ill, then lose her baby? You had a fear of childbearing and even though you didn't realize it, you have carried me all these years."
>
> As I stayed with this experience, I remembered that when I was thirty, I came to realize that this fear had been in me all these years, but I was too ashamed and embarrassed to tell anyone. Now as I lay on my bed, I held the fear, accepted it, cradled it in my arms. I said, "It's O.K. that you are part of me. I accept you and I don't ignore you anymore." The fear was changed somehow and this was a moment of grace and acceptance for me of my past fear which I continue to carry.

Three years before her surgery, this woman had begun to bleed excessively. Her doctor suspected menopause, which came as a shock to her. As she let in the significance of this movement toward physical infertility, she became aware that she was grieving:

Those three years of mourning or anticipatory grief were actually a gift to me. I began to really love my body — my whole self. So when I had the hysterectomy, I had in fact already grieved the loss of my childbearing parts of my body. . . . Yet there was something else there that needed to be acknowledged and accepted — the unconscious fear that I had for many years regarding the bearing of children. The "Focusing" was a big help to me in that it gave me a way to work with what was going on deep within me. Those three years of mourning the loss of my fertility, the actual surgery, and the "Focusing" experience were a real gift because I came to love myself — my whole self — in a new way. I came to appreciate my sexuality and all that it means to me as a celibate woman.

Many women who open themselves to the teaching of their bodies at this time of life find themselves led back to their premenstrual experience. Sometimes it comes from the years of the early teens, sometimes the latency age of nine through twelve, and sometimes it is the experience of the little girl who needs to be re-membered. One woman went through a period of many months considering her need for a hysterectomy. After gaining a sense that this was the right thing for her to do, and in preparation for her surgery, she found herself reconnecting with her little girl:

That free little girl who ran around in her underwear and played with the angels. . . . I'm feeling like that person I liked before I went to school. In order to get along on the playground, I took on a personality that made me popular. But now that girl in the garden is there with the grown-up me adding maturity and balance. I can take that combination into anything I do.

Remembering — whether it is through embracing, forgiving, accepting, or enjoying — is healing or whole-making, for it frees energy to join us where we are now and creates newness.

5. Grieving Our Losses

As women pilgrims on this journey through menopause, the chalice of the womb leads us to a new place through the process of our bodies' emptying. This is a process of letting go, this movement toward "zero ova," the emptying out of the fruit of our wombs, the ending of our time of physical fertility.

This movement is gradual for most of us, for some not fast enough, for others too soon, too fast. For some it is an eager countdown to zero and an anticipated celebration. Marge Piercy speaks of this in the last lines of her poem "Something to look forward to":

Today supine, groaning with demon crab claws
gouging my belly, I tell you I will secretly dance
and pour out a cup of wine on the earth

when time stops that leak permanently;
I will burn my last tampons as votive candles.[1]

For others there is a sense of loss and accompanying grief. A group of women were talking about their experience with menstruation as young girls and how that effects them in their approaching menopause. One woman, remembering that time of life through a journal exercise, spoke out with feeling: "I never realized how much I loved my period!" Later she reflected on her response:

> I was surprised to see how strongly I associated it with pleasurable things like childbearing, feeling womanly, etc. I'm sure that is in large part due to the way it was presented to me at the beginning, and I was also urged to be active and not curtail any athletic activity with that excuse — with the exception of swimming until I could use tampons.
>
> I guess I do unconsciously fear the loss, though I certainly would not want to have any more children now. Strange — as long as I continue to get my period, I guess I feel young, and I don't like the thought of getting old (frankly, I never imagined I *would* get old!).

Letting in the reality of this change, getting old, is sometimes the beginning of a grief process. For this active mid-life woman to no longer have her period meant a letting go of what had always given her a "young" and "womanly" feeling. As she stated her awareness, "I guess I do unconsciously fear the loss," she moved out of her denial, represented so honestly in her words, "Frankly, I never imagined I *would* get old!"

Denial, according to Elisabeth Kubler-Ross,[2] is the first stage in the grief process. Some of us do grieve the movement toward infertility in our bodies. Kubler-Ross's stages of grief clarify many of the feelings that some women have during this passage. The stages do not always follow in a linear order, but they do represent necessary phases in the movement through grief.

Denial

A vivacious forty-five-year-old wore sunglasses as she came into the building where the first workshop for "Women in Menopause" was held. She acknowledged on arrival that she didn't want people to know she was coming to the group. She told us that when she first read the article announcing the workshop, she exclaimed, "That's not me . . . that's my mother!" Then smiling, she said, "Of course, denial is the first stage of grief, isn't it?"

A woman who in her adult life developed arthritis spoke of her young self, "I was a tree climber. I loved to fly down stairs several at a time. Now I have to climb ladders so carefully at work. When I go downstairs, I can only go one step at a time. I fight this!" Coming to terms with our bodies' limitations is so difficult.

I had a similar experience a few years ago while working with a group of kids. My colleague and I joined their game of capture the flag. In the heat of the moment, as I saw him rushing toward jail to free his teammates, my forty-eight-year-old body hurled through the air to tag him as I would have forty years ago. I saved the day for our team but threw my back out. That's denial.

We don't want to accept these changes. We don't want to let go of what was. The grief process moves along when we acknowledge to ourselves and to others that we fight change. The woman who loved to climb trees and run down stairs described that wonderful feeling: "It was like flying — it seemed I *could* fly, just take off and soar." Letting go of that particular experience was grief for her. She finally recognized that she was continually pushing her body to do things faster and more freely than was possible for her at forty- nine. She was no longer denying that reality, even though there was sadness in letting be what was so. This response is not passive or submissive. It is a "Yes, this is so" versus a resistance to what is.

In the life passage of menopause, we are really facing our mortality, the fact that we do age and ultimately die. We may have thought about this fact, but our denial is often present. We say things like, "If I die, then I want you to have. . . ." There is no "if," there is only "when." It is no wonder that denial of our aging is the first stage of our grief.

Anger

"I never thought I'd be sitting on a park bench talking about losing my teeth. I'm wild! I need time. I have so much I want to do!" Losing some of her teeth was for this fifty-year-old woman symbolic of aging. It hit her in that instant as she expressed her anger. Her fuming and fire about teeth had to do with her sense of not having enough time to do what she wanted to do because she was getting old.

In our mothers' generation, outbursts like this were considered to be "erratic emotions" caused by the Change. Often no connection was made between the object of the anger, like teeth, and what was going on inside the woman — the understandable frustration of facing limitations at a time when she felt eager to get on with her life.

In our mothers' day, people who expressed anger freely were often labeled "bitchy," or "so emotional," and sometimes they were thought to be "going crazy with the Change." It is not surprising that many of that generation tried to be "stoic," as one mid-life woman recalls. They would "minimize their feelings, which in the long run may not have been helpful to others. I'm not sure how constructive it was for them either." She also recognized the modeling that it provided for her as a woman. "Even now I am often uncomfortable after I've let my feelings out. I feel foolish and exposed."

A woman who had her career before having children at thirty was currently planning, at fifty, on her children moving out so she could be "free." Her son decided to commute to school and live at home. Her response was anger: "I feel a sense of urgency about getting on with *my* life, discovering what I can do. I don't want to waste my time. I want to get on with it." She found herself often expressing anger toward her son, anger that she recognized as only a part of what was actually going on. Her frustration was with her life circumstances that were not coinciding with her inner sense of "now it is my time, and time is moving on."

Anger often covers deeper feelings. I learned this from an unforgettable experience. A friend of mine committed suicide in the late summer. I was devastated by her death. At the time I didn't realize it, but I became very depressed. I would often overreact to a situation in my own life and blow off about it. I felt like a loose cannon careening across a ship's deck, exploding in various directions as the ship moved in stormy waters.

It took eight weeks for me to finally explode at God and then at my friend for taking her own life. I let it rip like never before. And then I really felt the sadness of my loss. In retrospect I realize that my anger was directed appropriately toward God and my friend, but it also carried intense firepower from my own fear of losing *my* life, of dying inside.

A few years earlier I had expressed those fears in my journal:

Am I willing to die?
    asks the hollow-wombed woman
    the dry-breasted woman
    the dying woman

Am I willing to release my grasp on life?
Am I willing to stop trying to make it better?
Am I willing to let be what is?

Am I willing to give up the illusion
    that I created
    these children of mine?

Am I willing to die
    in order to have new life?

Beneath my anger and fear was the sadness that I was feeling over letting go of my children whose lives were moving them on and away. This external life change often occurs around the time that we are becoming aware of our move toward infertility. Feelings like mine used to be labeled as signs of depression with a capital D. Our feelings are a legitimate part of the grief process. Feelings need to be expressed in a place that is safe. A journal offers that kind of safety as a starting place for expression. Sharing the feelings, recognizing their significance helps to move us on in the grief process.

Bargaining

A woman who is a health practitioner, whose lifework is dedicated to assisting others toward well-being, recognized her way of bargaining with the signs of her approaching menopause and thus the signs of her mortality. She heard herself saying to herself, "If I walk and swim, eat well, meditate, go on retreats, and daily say an affirmation about my well-being, then I won't have those signs of aging: I won't need glasses. I won't need a D&C. I won't have to go through those things that I hear others talking about." She became aware that she was bargaining.

My own fear of osteoporosis has often driven my routine of walking and swimming. Exercising regularly and eating well, I have been determined not to develop porous bones. A similar kind of bargaining effort may lie behind our society's frantic efforts to stay in shape. The pharmaceutical companies play on the fear of aging that lies behind this hyperactivity with their bargaining approach in the advertising of hormone replacement therapy. They claim that if you take hormones, then "The Change of Life doesn't have to change yours," as an ad for one product says.[3]

We may choose hormone therapy to assist us in this rebalancing process if the benefits to us as an individual outweigh the known risks. However, if we choose to make this choice, it is healthier to acknowledge whatever is actually happening rather than pretending that there will be no changes. The desire to believe that aging will not happen tempts everyone, but that bargain is not possible. So we often experience anger and sadness when we finally take in the signs of our mortality.

Depression

Keeping our feelings of fear, anger, or sadness about our mortality inside is a way that we can depress ourselves. I learned this the hard way by not expressing myself for six weeks after my friend's suicide. Irene Stiver and Jean Baker Miller also note that "depressive periods" are experienced by "twice as many women as men," with "married women in particular . . . more prone to develop depressions than both married men or single women who are heads of households."[4] Many married women look to their spouses for a level of intimacy and understanding that is not possible in that relationship because many men have not learned how to express or deal with feelings:

> Our basic notion is that many women who suffer depression have not been able to experience their sadness, and most important, have not been able to experience it within a context of empathic and validating relationships. There is one major reason why this occurs: the people in the surrounding context of relationships (and often in society in general) do not recognize that a disappointment or loss occurred. Alternately, they may recognize that some kind of loss has occurred, but they do not recognize its significance or magnitude for the woman.[5]

We now do have opportunities to be in or to create contexts where our feelings are received and others seek to understand the significance or magnitude of our losses. This makes it possible, for example, to move from expressing anger about losing teeth or about kids' unpredictability, to expressing sadness about lost opportunities. We can recognize with each other that these losses *are* significant and that the magnitude does differ with individual experience. We can and must do this for each other.

A male spouse or partner cannot know the experience of menopause, nor can a male psychotherapist through clinical observation, nor a young female doctor just because she is female. Even we ourselves who are in this passage cannot know exactly the level of sadness in another's loss. We can, however, provide a context in which we encourage one another to express our feelings of grief and loss. In doing this we validate each other's experience.

In one group, a woman who had been feeling depressed began to talk about how she had recently started saying "No" to her husband's and children's assumptions regarding what she would do for them. We acknowledged the conflict that she was creating beween their and her own "good wife" and "good mother" expectations. Her family awoke one morning to find Post-it notes all over the house, saying, "No! I won't put your dirty clothes away!" "No! You may not take my keys to use the car this morning!" "No! I will not make your lunch!" etc.

As she acknowledged to the group these late-night declarations, we could feel the explosion of energy released when she connected with her anger and then with her sadness at her loss of self. We understood and applauded her expression. We heard her into recognizing the magnitude of this loss. Having been heard, she could begin to express the self that wanted to come forth in her own right.

Shifting from depression to expression is what moves us on in the grief process.

Acceptance

Remember the woman who loved to climb trees as a young girl, who especially liked flying up and down stairs, for whom running felt like soaring? This same person, at forty-eight, after a day of hard physical work, with her body now aching from arthritis, found that even climbing the stairs to her bedroom was labor. Pushing herself to exercise, blaming herself for not being able to move freely, trying all kinds of therapies to bargain against her changing body, she felt anger at herself, her heredity, her situation. She experienced depression.

Then she allowed herself to feel her sadness over the loss of that playful agility. She allowed herself to grieve. She began to accept what was so in her life, to let be what was. She let there be that sense of loss, that emptiness. She began to let go and let be.

In that deep spiritual movement of acceptance, she opened herself to something new. She came to realize that her mind could still take off and fly. She has a wonderful, inquisitive mind that in fact soars and plays with new ideas. She recognized that the same tomboy quality was alive and well within her. While she still needs to be very mindful of her body's limitations, she can play with ideas in a free-spirited, delightful way.

For this woman and for all of us who are moving through the stages from denial to acceptance, letting go is the theme. I have felt this most powerfully in my own on-going relationship with physical limitations. With each new area of change, I have fought the truth of my body's feedback. I am slowly learning that my body holds deep wisdom for me with which I can cooperate. Letting go of the way it was and moving into the way it is now is not a once-and-for-all process. We all go back and feel again the desire to deny what is so. We try to make deals with our body. We reexperience the anger and depression that comes as we slowly move toward letting go and acceptance.

Grieving our losses is an emptying process. When we open ourselves to this process, we can see that it is also a part of our journey into the unknown of a new phase of life. This time of not-knowing is sometimes experienced as being without a sense of purpose. There is an emptiness that previously we have been able to fill. Staying with that emptiness, like staying with the emptying process of our womb, is not easy. However, it can be a deeply spiritual time. Other pilgrims have made their way through to a "place of the break-through into abundance."[6] Their experience encourages us in our journey toward the new.

6. Allowing Empty Space

In the Middle Ages people believed that if there ever was a blank or empty space, the Devil would rush in to fill it up. When a person sneezed, it was thought that a vacuum was created. Therefore another person should quickly say, "God bless you!" to fill that empty space and keep the Devil out. Our Puritan forebears carried this fear forward into daily life with their work ethic, which kept hands and minds always busy. Empty space, like darkness, was threatening. Quick, fill it up!

It is hard to open ourselves to a different experience of emptiness and darkness with these and other more contemporary fears in our psyches. Many of us know painful feelings and images that return to us when there is empty space, when we are not doing something. We dread those feelings or memories. We seek to avoid their pain. Darkness, too, for many women has held extremely painful experiences. Around our country women have been moving to "take back the night," to reclaim safety for each other and all people in the darkness. We also need to reclaim and rename the experience of personal darkness. Our bodies' process at menopause gives us the opportunity to know emptiness and darkness as empty space.

In many spiritual traditions, including the Judeo-Christian heritage, creation came out of nothing, and "darkness covered the face of the deep" (Gen. 1:2). German mystic Meister Eckhart spoke of the ground of the soul as dark. Our own lives began in the rich and nourishing environment of the womb's darkness. The germination of a seed takes place in the darkness of the soil. Life, miraculous life, begins in darkness. The bulb replenishes underground in the winter's dark soil.

We are much more at ease with summer's light. We can learn from those who have come to love the winter. An older woman expressed her need for darkness in Judith Duerk's *Circle of Stones*:

> It was only when I lived through the summer solstice light, far above the Arctic Circle, the light of the longest day in our year, the totality of white, white, ever-pervasive light, day after day, that I experienced our desperate need for darkness, for shadow, for relief from the clarity, sharpness, and rationality that this present world demands. . . .
>
> Now, winter returns, the darkness . . . the year, come full circle again . . . a chance, again, to sink into one's own stillness . . . a time to feel one's fatigue, the aches of life, one's own age, to reconnect, once again, with a deep, dark, earth-energy, hidden far below in our roots.[1]

When we do open ourselves to the rhythms of nature, our own and that of all creation, we experience a balancing movement. As we venture in this time of life to experience our *own* experience, we can open ourselves to learning from the rhythms of our wombs once again. Replenishing and shedding, filling and emptying, fullness and emptiness are the movements that we have known since we became women. We know this natural balancing rhythm in our bodies as life's cycle. The interaction of these apparent opposites becomes a creative interplay from which new life can emerge. When we allow ourselves to experience both the light and the darkness, the full and the empty, then the creative process occurs. Creation involves both.

I first learned about empty space through the process of being emptied. I would not have chosen this first teacher, but physical pain taught me that, like a bucket, I could not be filled until I was emptied. In my early forties, before I understood that I needed to pace myself, I injured my back. A series of factors had been piled one on top of the other over the years, stress being the common fluid that ran through them all. One day I added the final twist to that column.

My body's response was spasm and sciatica. I spent six months on my back, the first fourteen days lying on the floor in the living room of our home. My only trips during those days were to the bathroom. The doorways in our old house had thresholds. Each time I was assisted over those two-inch thresholds, I felt effort in my body as if I were ascending Mount Everest. In the following days and weeks and months of various kinds of beds, exercises, adjustments, prescriptions, reading everything that I could, receiving advice, and seeking all kinds of assistance, I worked hard to heal myself. The pain would not be relieved.

tears, screams, fists against the wall . . .
sobs, shouts, groaning from within.

I can't! I can't! I can't! I can't!
I've tried so hard and I can't make it be better!

I remember that day and my utter frustration with what seemed to be *zero* results — nothing was changing, just pain, recurring pain.

At some point, I felt myself stop making the effort, as though I had finally taken a deep breath and then let the air out slowly. I stopped trying so hard. I stopped pushing myself to heal. I let go. And then slowly it dawned on me: The healing was taking place in the spaces between my efforts. The healing was taking place in the empty space. I needed to trust that. I could not choose whether or not I had pain, but by letting go and letting myself be, I could choose to empty myself of my effort and open myself to the healing that was taking place in the empty space.

Letting pain be pain has not been our society's idea of a good thing. This applies to emotional pain as well as to physical pain. "I haven't got time for the pain" may translate into something like "I don't want to deal with the pain. Just help me get rid of it!" Yet experience has taught me and others with whom I work that the journey with the pain and the ultimate letting go does give us new energy. It can have a transforming effect on our lives. One woman told me,

> In the good old days I did what I had been explicitly taught by my family, teachers, and culture: move away from pain. Use aspirin, other drugs, television, alcohol, high sensation things, "love," anything that will "help the pain go away." No one ever suggested that pain has a wonderful function: telling me exactly where healing is needed and why!
>
> Through the "Focusing" method I have learned first, that it is safe to feel pain; second, that pain is more painful when I don't feel it; and third, that simply feeling the pain is quite often the remedy for whatever ails me. Old pain persists because when I was a child, certain events were unbearable and not feeling them enabled a kind of survival. That survival allows me now the opportunity to return to flags of declarant pain and to process the experiences held there with my current resources.
>
> Gradually I have learned that I have an alternative to fearing pain, and I can recognize pain now as yet one more part of the miraculous equipment of life. With experience I now have confidence that feeling the pain — when I'm ready — is the first step in a healing process that my being already knows about. The process is put into effect by taking that first step. Feeling the pain has helped me move from the isolation of denial to the healing of being.

These are the words of a woman who is approaching menopause and like many has found a heightened sense of memory during this life passage. Through the "Focusing" technique, she has found a way to take time with the pain, enabling her to make her journey from the isolation of denial, through the empty space of not-knowing, to the healing of being.

Choosing to empty oneself is different from being emptied by the experience of trauma or physical pain. It takes courage to consciously allow empty space to be empty space. It is not easy. A friend who had been extremely active and creative as a psychothera-pist, wife, mother, and friend experienced a deep loss. At fifty she was finding it very difficult to let herself grieve, to let pain be pain, and to be in the darkness of not-knowing. She knew well the opposite in her activity, busyness, and "creating crisis," as she put it. This had always filled the vacuum. It was scary for her to begin to let there be a vacuum, an empty space. "Don't just stand there, *do* something!" were the words that rang in her ears, and in mine now as I remember her saying, "But that's what I grew up on!" Even so there was an attraction at this time in her life to discovering what empty space might be like.

She began to experiment with allowing empty space to be there and tried not to fill it up. She described this when she said, "I am sinking into my own stillness." Sinking into this quiet darkness felt like a dying to the busy, fearful part of herself. She began to experience this emptiness, not as a vacuum, but as a time of waiting, a gestation period. I reflected on this in a poem:

> The death of the panicky self
> > becomes a seed
> > falling into darkness
> The darkness
> > becomes the place
> > of patient nurturing
> The seed
> > becomes the source
> > of creativity

> The seed in the fallow field
> nurtured in quiet depths,
> a balance to creative expansion,
> . . . patient nurturing.

As she ventured in this way, she also learned from other women of their need for solitude at this time in their lives. As one person said, "It's different from being the loner of long ago. Now you go to solitude."

Another woman spoke of her need: "I need lots of solitude. When you are alone, you can be the new stuff. You don't fall back into old patterns." She acknowledged at the same time the need for interconnection, but she had a sense that emptiness allowed space for newness to be experienced. Sometimes "old stuff" does come up. "My fear of being a wallflower comes back," a woman acknowledged to a group who were talking about empty space. "So when I connect with those painful years, I just let myself sit with and be with what is. [Doing that,] I now experience a clarity that has come to me a lot."

Meditation is one way in which we can choose to cooperate with our emptying process. It takes discipline or desire to let go into empty space, to let silence be Silence, to be receptive and wait in the darkness of not-knowing. We can learn how to make space within through a simple daily practice. The word "meditation" is used in many ways. The following distillation represents a way that I find very helpful:

> Sit down. Sit still and upright. Keep your eyes slightly open, allowing your gaze to fall unfocused about three feet in front of you. Sit relaxed and alert.
>   Silently, interiorly begin to say a single word joined with your inhalation or exhalation or both.

Depending on your spiritual tradition or your individual choice, the word needs to provide a focus but is most effective if its meaning does not engage your conscious mind. When you have selected a word or, as is often the case, the word selects you, "sound it gently but continuously in your heart," letting go of "all thought of its meaning."

"Do not imagine anything — spiritual or otherwise. When thoughts, feelings, and images come up, let them come and let them go. Just return again to simply saying the word in the depths of your being."[2]

There are many times when it is impossible to clear the space. Feelings, plans, ideas keep coming into our minds. It can be helpful to have a pad of paper beside you as you meditate to write down the things that pull for your attention. Putting them on paper enables you temporarily to let them go and not hold them in that inner space. It is also helpful to have someone — a counselor, clergy person, spiritual guide, or friend — to work with or talk to about the hard, confusing, or painful things that sometimes come up in the empty space.

This particular way of meditation has deep roots in the Christian tradition, as well as being central to some Eastern spiritual traditions. There are many good books and articles available to help support this practice. A growing number of resources can be found that encourage meditation for the recovery of health and the maintenance of personal well-being.

To sit with painful things that come up in the emptiness or darkness is not comfortable. However, the practice of meditation encourages our ability to let things come and let them go, once again the rhythm of holding and shedding. To sit in this way means to allow the feelings, thoughts, and images to come but not to hold onto them or follow them. Rather, the rhythm is like breathing or the movement of a wave on the beach — coming in and going out — washing through the space of our being.

Once I wrote of my own longing to let go into this empty space:

Sinking into God —
Go back to the beginning:
   before all action,
      before all proving,
         before all needing,
            before all longing,
               before all separation,
                  before all aloneness,
                    before all fear.

As any one who meditates knows, this is much easier said than done. It involves a deep level of trust, which threatens our survival instincts and thus our controlling mind.

As a child of nine I almost drowned, pulled by the powerful undertow of Lake Michigan. I wore glasses then, so without them the shoreline was blurry. I knew my friend had gone for help, but I could not see anyone. The waves were high. I have a visceral memory of my struggle to stay on top, to get my breath, fighting not to go under. At that time I did not know that the best thing to do was to go with the undertow, to let go into it. The bodily memory of my panic still gets touched off in situations where what is needed is to let go. Even though I still love to swim, the words "sinking into God" challenge my willingness to trust. So my mind often reaches for all manner of thoughts and images to keep a sense of control, to resist letting go and resting in the emptiness.

There are other ways to empty oneself, to let go of thoughts, images, plans, or "crises" that crowd our minds and lives. There are different ways to empty that inner space. For some, immersing oneself in water, wind, or natural beauty does this. Exercising physically until one is spent gives a bodily sense of emptiness. Sex, with its rhythm of heightened sensation until orgasm and rest, is a way in which we can experience this kind of cleared space. It is also experienced by some people after a time of total absorption in a creative act that concludes with a catharsis when the creation comes forth. An empty space often follows.

I am slowly learning that we do not need to fear empty space as a threat to life. Some of us may still experience the fears of our Puritan forebears. We may still feel the lingering effects of that fear when we hear older female friends and relatives say about the Change of life, "Just keep busy, and you'll get through it." It is my experience, and the experience of many of the women with whom I have worked, that we can do more than just get through it. We can choose to move with the emptying rhythm of our bodies. We can learn from nature's wisdom about the balancing process of emptying and filling. This conscious journey through menopause in cooperation with our bodies can lead us to a new place.

Traveling to this new place, we do often go through darkness and not-knowing. We encounter unfamiliar territory; we discover empty space. Like cartographers who call blank spaces on a map "sleeping beauties,"[3] we, too, can envision potential in the unknown. Annie Dillard, whose poetic prose often reaches beyond words to direct experience, is one who empties herself and is emptied by her oneness with the natural world. In reflecting on the polar explorers and on her own expedition into that land of "sleeping beauties" and blizzards' white emptiness, she describes the part of the spiritual journey explored in this chapter, the movement into empty space:

> You walk, and one day you enter the spread heart of silence, where land dissolves and sea becomes vapor and ices sublime under unknown stars. This is the land of the Via Negativa, the lightless edge where the slopes of knowledge dwindle, and love for its own sake, lacking an object, begins.[4]

7. Letting Go
. . . to
Embrace

Flowing red out of my body
    I know what it is!
    I'm not a boy!
    I'm a girl
        a girl
        a girl
    I am going to be . . .
        I'm going to be . . .
                someday a woman.

I am a woman
I bleed each month
    right on time
I feel the filling up of me until, until, until . . .
    I let it go

The letting go feels
    deep in my womb place
    a soreness yet a joy!
       I am a woman.

The rhythm of filling up and emptying, shedding and replenishing, is our womb's gift to us. We can know with a bodily knowing what it is to feel fullness and what it is to let go.

As young girls we experienced this for the first time through our menses, but most of us at that time were not very conscious of the natural rhythm that connects us with all creation and Life itself. Those who have borne children, watched them grow, and then go on their way have known that same rhythm of fullness and emptiness. As we approach menopause, we can experience the emptying and filling in a new way.

The movement toward barrenness and the empty space of winter and then the coming of new life and the promise of spring is a profound spiritual movement. This feminine rhythm is recognized through the myth of Persephone and Demeter, which speaks of the connection between mother and daughter. In its earliest version, Demeter, the Grain Mother Goddess, and Persephone, the Grain Maiden, had an abundant life together and were beloved by mortals. Demeter gave them the gift of wheat. Persephone enjoyed her life as a maiden of the fields, but she became concerned about the spirits of the dead mortals who seemed lost. She decided to go to the underworld to assist them. Her mother did not want her to leave, but Persephone persisted. She left her mother to descend to the underworld, carrying three poppies and three sheaves of her mother's grain.[1] Demeter's grief over the absence of her daughter was so great that the Goddess of Grain forbade all new growth. The earth lay barren.

After months of bleakness, one day Demeter's grief was penetrated by a sign of new life pushing through the ground. She knew that this could only be a sign of Persephone's return. Her joy was so great, as she spread the good news, that new life began to push forth everywhere. When Demeter saw Persephone coming up from the underworld, she ran to her and they embraced.

Letting go is not something that even a Mother Goddess does easily, much less we mortals. We do feel our loss, and we need to grieve in the process of letting go. Grieving is real and necessary for true change to occur. For if we do not experience totally the letting go, with its accompanying grief, we often create real conflict and pain for ourselves as we try to hold on to what has been.

This can be especially true in relation to one's last child. In my case it was my youngest daughter. Re-membering my connection with her helped in understanding my own difficulty in letting go. Her birth was critical. Near the end of the delivery, a nurse noticed a low fetal heartbeat and realized that the umbilical cord was being pinched. My husband, Cam, was sent out of the room. It was rare in those days for husbands to be allowed to stay through a delivery. Little did they know the support he gave me through his constant prayer in the minutes that followed.

"You've got twenty minutes to get that baby out!" I was told. Within that atmosphere of urgency, I had a sense of being protected from fear as if I were surrounded by a plastic bubble. All my energy was free to move with my body. When my daughter came out, I had an overwhelming sense of relief and gratitude, which Cam and I shared.

Later when I was taken to my room, I began to realize just how critical the situation had been. As my mind took hold of that reality, I wound myself up into an extreme high, which lasted throughout the days in the hospital. At one point I remember feeling that I was the Queen of Heaven. I could look down and see the whole planet earth lying beneath me. I had never experienced anything like that before. It took several days after I came home to come down from that birth experience. My husband helped me in simple ways by cutting stimulation from light and sounds, playing Mozart, reminding me to focus on my breathing and to stay in the here-and-now. Slowly I became grounded again.

Our daughter's birth was a powerful experience for me. However, in the days that followed, as I reflected on the aftermath, I became scared. I wanted to understand what had happened and how I could have been so far "out there." I asked my gynecologist what he thought about my postpartum experience. He never gave me an answer. I asked various other "experts" over time. Most of them did not want to explore it. So I tried not to dwell on what had happened to me or to get close to that kind of edge again.

During the time of my passage through menopause, I have been re-membering important events in my life. In doing so, I have come to a deeper understanding of that birth experience, which I used to fear had pushed me over the edge into craziness and might happen again. As I trust my own experience more, I am now able to claim that event as a truly sacred moment in time and beyond time. I have the sense that the life-and-death intensity of that birth experience opened me to Mystery and a moment of oneness with the Great Mother, the Queen of Heaven.

As I now let this deep knowing surface, I have had a sense of "Yes, that is so!" The gift of this awareness adds to my understanding of the difficulty that I have in letting go of my role as mother.

When our first child left, I came to a very helpful realization. I became aware that when children finally go out the door (although the current generation, in this time of economic squeeze, tends to use what *Boston Globe* columnist Ellen Goodman has called a "revolving door"), we do feel their absence. We feel the absence of the quality or qualities that they added to our lives.

I noticed this first when our son left for a semester in Latin America. I missed him deeply. I missed his adventuresome mind, his stimulating questions. He is a learner. I grieved the loss of his presence in my life. Then I realized that his qualities that I missed so much were also in me. They were aspects of myself that I had not been developing or sharing. The learner in me responded to the learner in him. That awareness led me to involve myself in some in-depth study that rekindled my own inner student.

When our oldest daughter was in her senior year in high school, I began grieving. I anticipated the loss of her comforting presence and companionship. (I have since learned that the word "comfort" comes from the Latin meaning "with strength.") I have always loved being with her, no matter what we were doing. When she did leave, I realized that I also had a nurturing part of myself that needed to be expressed. I began to put energy into baking, making soup, and enjoying our home as a place of comfort and hospitality.

As our youngest child was preparing to move away to start her first job, I again did some grieving ahead of time. I recorded an awareness about my mourning process in my journal: "That is what I have been grieving — losing her vitality. She is full of life. I fear the loss of that in myself as I move into this next chapter of life. My children have been my fruit and signs of being fully alive."

Later I was helped by a powerful dream:

I find a baby that has been hidden in the closet for a long time. She has signs of fully developed breasts, but her legs are not yet developed. I have forgotten about her because so much is going on. She is wrapped up in a small white box. She is not alive. I feel great grief.

It was the kind of dream that at first I wanted to forget. I also knew from experience that however painful it was, the dream had come from the place of deep knowing. I needed to pay attention to it. Through the disturbing image in this dream, I realized that there was a new life within waiting to be developed. The dream felt like a call from my deep self to no longer hide away the life that has been given to me. Keeping it in the closet was truly anti-life.

Reflecting on the dream, I wrote in my journal:

I am being called to attention. I cannot keep my vitality — my love of life — in the closet. It will die. That life needs to be tended and out in the light to fully develop. It has to do with being a fully developed woman. It would be a great loss if I kept this in the closet. . . . There is more to come. I need to develop legs (supports) to help me in being full of life.

The ending of my central role as mother had connected me with something very important. As I realized how I had been holding on to that part of my life, I also gained more understanding of my own mother. This mother-daughter connection is certainly powerful for those who are related by birth. As Adrienne Rich has said in *Of Woman Born*, "The materials are here for the deepest mutuality and the most painful estrangement."[2] For those who come to this relationship out of choice — through adoption or stepparenting — or out of necessity — taking on the roles of mother or daughter in difficult circumstances — the connection develops over time. All of us have our individual stories and images of this relationship.

Rosario Morales used the image of the umbilical cord to express her experience of "mutuality" with her daughter, with whom she was collaborating in writing a book:

> This book began in long budget-breaking phone calls stretched across the width of this country . . . through the good times and the bad, the fights and the making up, the long sullen silences and the happy chatter cluttering the phone lines strung between us like a 3,000-mile umbilical cord from navel to navel, mine to hers, hers to mine, each of us mother and daughter by turns, feeding each other the substance of our dreams.[3]

The mother-daughter cord is there for all of us. Whether it is knotted, tangled, or clear; whether it carries nourishment, anger, or static, the connection is there. Often we have to let go of old ways of connecting in order to make space for new ways to emerge. Even when there has been painful estrangement, most mothers and daughters "hang in there," according to Janet Surrey in a lecture on mother-daughter issues in psychotherapy. Hanging in there

> is not evidence of stuck, unresolved relationships, although sometimes it feels that way, but rather evidence of courage, stamina, persistence, loyalty, and commitment.

. . . So most of us hang in there and it gets a little better.
There are some predictable changes by age, marital status,
and the fact that both mothers and daughters today have
new opportunities for growth and development. Perhaps
conflict and misunderstanding are inevitable.[4]

As older daughters approaching our menopause, we have the
opportunity to follow the wisdom of our changing bodies as we grow
and develop in this third phase of our lives. For as we experience the
movement of letting go on a bodily level, we can also be aware that
the same spiritual movement may need to develop in our relationships.

Janice Mirikitani acknowledges how hard it is to let go of the old
ways of relating in her dedication "For My Daughter" in the poem
"Sing With Your Body":

We love with great difficulty
spinning in one place
afraid to create
        spaces
            new rhythm . . . [5]

We may find as mothers and as daughters that the movement of
letting go at this time of life enables us to create spaces and find a new
rhythm in our relationships that heretofore had not seemed possible.
This has been true for me.

My mother is a strong, creative, intelligent, and socially concerned woman who has been my model for wife, mother, and
minister's wife. This triple-decker assignment has intensified the
kinds of expectations that I placed on her and myself. As many
daughters do, I tried to be like her, and then I tried to be unlike her.
I held her ways as a standard, and I also reacted against them. I wanted
her to support me as I grew to be a woman, and I pushed her away.
I swore I would never marry a minister, and I did. I compared myself
with her in many ways, and I often devalued myself in so doing. I

learned the pain of comparison. Throughout my twenties and thirties I felt ambivalence toward my mother as I tried to find my own way into those roles that we both played.

When I compared myself with my mother (and with other strong women), I often held back on what I was experiencing. Because our strengths are different, I often withheld my more intuitive, feeling way of perceiving things. I was awed by her quick mind and verbal skills, so I would hold back on what I felt, what I knew from my own experience, what was mine to share. I began to feel like a bird who was withholding her own song because it was not as beautiful, brilliant, or exciting as that of another. Over time this withholding separated me from life, from others, from my mother, and from my true self.

I became aware of this suppressed energy through my body's tension and subsequent pain. I realized that withholding my own life energy in certain relationships was a real denial of the life that is uniquely mine, and I was the one who was paying the price. The loss was mine, and now I see that it was a loss for others, too. Through therapy, journal work, reflection with others, and the events of my life, I came to realize that I needed to let go of comparing myself with my mother. This involved letting go of the picture of her that I had been holding onto very tightly.

In releasing my grasp on the way I saw things, I had to begin to look at what was actually so, to learn what my mother's life was really like — her girlhood, her young womanhood, her hopes, dreams, and longings. As I listened, really listened with my heart, to her story, I began to take in the shyness that she covers so well, her pain, and the things that really bring her joy. I began to allow her to be to me who she really was all along. I was then able to appreciate her and truly to see her in the chapter of life that she is currently living. It was very exciting and releasing.

My mother and father moved to a new community after Dad retired from the parish ministry. For a ten-year period my mother was very active in peace and justice work. Beginning in her late sixties, she took leadership roles with a singleness of purpose that she had never had time to do before. My father took the self-named role of househusband and was very supportive of her work. We spent time together in the summers, and I came to love and appreciate her artistic nature, her love of poetry, especially that of Emily Dickinson. It was during this time that I came to see my mother as another person who was truly singing her own song:

Bright eyes sparkling
        within a wrinkled face
once smooth skin sacrificed
        to living and to loving
small creature quickness
        of body, mind, and spirit
seizing an idea
        chewing and digesting it
        giving it to her young
                and others,
holding back less and less
        her convictions and judgments,
she clarifies herself
        as she initiates.

How far you've come
        from Emily's retirement
        to yours
        the poetry remembered still
        and with your own
        merges
        as lines come up to greet
        a sunset
        or the dawn.

Sing on
        your song
        for it is your song to sing.

As I finished writing this poem in my journal, the tears came. I had a sense of a great letting go, and in that letting go a space opened up for me to embrace not only my mother but also myself. As I let go of my way of seeing and comparing, I not only saw and heard my mother in a new way, I also released some powerful energy that had been stuck between us. It was available to me in a new way as an encouragement to discover and to create that which was truly *my* song, the song that I alone could sing.

III. Drinking Deeply

8. Knowing and Choosing

My mother had an expression that stayed with me especially when I was a young mother because I found it very difficult to live it out. She would say, "When you assent, assent gladly. When you refuse, refuse definitely." I translated this to mean, "Let your Yes be Yes, and let your No be No."

It is so easy to waffle in between with an "Oh, all right" that sounds and feels like a Yes/No. The energy of a Yes/No is often halfhearted and, therefore, does not feel good. It feels more like a burden that is taken on than a choice that is made.

I think there is real wisdom in my mother's saying. I also think it takes a lot of self-knowledge to be able to make a Yes be Yes. Perhaps that is why it worked for my mother as a mature woman and not so well for me as a young mother. I remember finally figuring out that if the kids came to me with a request that I just could not handle, wanting an answer *Now*, I would say, "I'm going to the bathroom to think about it. I'll tell you my answer when I come out." Sometimes I would stay in there a very long time. I think, however, that was a step in self-knowledge. I needed space to gather my thoughts. I do not work well under pressure.

As mature women, we now have the opportunity to clarify our choices based on our accumulated self-knowledge. A few years ago I was with a group of women who were discussing menopause and some of the benefits of moving toward maturity. We played with the idea that learning to say No was much deeper than an assertion of our self. It is essential to say No to some things in order to say Yes to the things that connect us with an expression of our true selves.

The group carried this a step further, applying it to Frederick Nietzsche's idea of "a sacred 'No'" and "a sacred 'Yes.'" We decided that in our life passage, with the harvest of our experience and self-knowledge, we have what it takes to make choices in a fuller way than in our earlier life. We can speak from what that group called *a sacred Know.*

In *Thus Spake Zarathustra*, Nietzsche spoke about "the three metamorphoses of the spirit . . . how the spirit becomes a camel; and the camel becomes a lion; and the lion, finally, becomes a child."[1] We can do some new naming from his understanding of the human spirit's journey. The camel we know well. It represents the dutiful one: "The spirit that would bear much takes upon itself" the burdens of others. That one finally "speeds into the desert."

In the desert, the emptiness, "the second metamorphosis occurs: here the spirit becomes a lion who would conquer his freedom and be master in his own desert." In the desert the lion realizes that it is the "great dragon" who has enslaved him. And his name is "Thou shalt." "But the spirit of the lion says, 'I will.'" To move from the burden of "I should" to the choice of "I will" takes lion or lioness energy.

However, the final stage takes a different kind of energy:
To create new values — that even the lion cannot do; but the creation of freedom for oneself for new creation — that

is within the power of the lion. . . . What can the child do that even the lion cannot do? Why must the preying lion still become a child? The child is innocence and forgetting, a new beginning, a game, a self-propelled wheel, a first movement, a sacred "Yes." For the game of creation . . . a sacred "Yes" is needed.[2]

When we name *our* experience, we recognize the creative back and forth movement that takes place between the sacred No and the sacred Yes. We do not move through a simple three-stage "metamorphosis," using the pioneer wagon-leader approach. The way we use our lioness energy in the on-going process of saying the sacred No is very important. Many women cannot just say No to duty or burdens that are theirs to bear. It is not that simple. A single parent, a woman caring for an elderly relative, or a grandmother becoming a parent to her daughter's child cannot simply throw up her hands, roar "I've had it!" and walk out without repercussions within herself.

Many of us have spent time in the desert facing the great dragon and his shoulds, wrestling with our sense of duty, and what feels like irreconcilable longings, hopes, and dreams. These desert times sometimes involve leaving those we love behind for a time, maybe hours, maybe days. A few months after the birth of our third child, I was overwhelmed with all the aspects of my life as a young mother. I felt a desperate need for some empty space. With my husband's support, I took off with my nursing baby to a community that welcomed people in emotional crisis. I had a room of my own and time to reflect. I continue to do this periodically by going on retreat. We need the empty space of the desert to gain our perspective. The desert can be any place where we encounter ourselves in a space set apart from our on-going life.

In spiritual writings throughout the centuries, "the desert" has always meant just that kind of empty space. For it is there, in the empty space, that we often touch our deeper knowing and then connect with the lioness spirit that moves us from "I should" to "I will." This movement to real choice enables us to pick up our duty, perhaps in a new way. Speaking from an "I will" rather than an "I should" comes from the sacred Know of self-knowledge more than the sacred No of self-determination.

Edith Sullwold, a Jungian therapist, was approaching her sixtieth birthday. She was very much aware that this particular year was recognized among the Chinese as the most important year in a woman's life. It is the year of the second commitment. The earlier years of a woman's life involve outer commitments. Then at sixty an inner commitment is made to spiritual depth and the wisdom of eldership.

Edith received a birthday card from an eighty-year-old friend. When she opened the card, sixty tiny pieces of purple paper fell out, each bearing the single word "No" on it. Her older friend was trying to give her a message about making too many commitments. She thought about it and came up with this response:

> I do not want to just say No flatly. I have decided that when I do not want to do something, after giving it consideration, I will say something like this: I think that is a very good (or interesting, challenging, creative, or whatever) idea. At this time in my life, however, it is not appropriate for me to do it.

A statement like this comes from the sacred Know. That source can feed the knowledge of our capabilities and limitations, which then becomes the basis for our choices as to where to direct our life energy. The No that comes from this deep source leads to a clearer Yes. There is great liberation in that kind of self-knowledge. The harvest of Edith's life and her work with adults and children comes from having journeyed deeply. Her pilgrimage has enabled her to speak from the sacred Know. She shares this journey both as a friend and as a master teacher of other therapists.

The sacred Know depends on the kind of traveling that the storyteller models. It is spiral in its course. The process of self-knowledge involves a circling back to pick up, re-member, and include what has come before. What has been informs what is now and what is to be. This connected inclusion enables us to experience a fuller sense of ourselves and adds richness to the harvest of our knowledge. It adds to the clarity of our choices as we move into the next season of our lives.

One woman expressed very well the cost of making choices: "Clarity comes when we pay attention to our living. Having a physical disability made me look at options. Do I want to paint, or do I want to be a mother? We all have to make choices. The choices are limiting, and the limits are enhancing." Another woman added, "I always thought that I would have a child. I chose not to have a child alone, not just to follow the biological urge. It was a moment-to-moment decision. If conditions had been right, my choice would have been different." Making choices from a place of self-knowledge, with "attention to our living," enables our choices to come from the sacred Know. When this is so, our choices, though limiting, enhance our true life.

I am aware that as a younger mother, I often responded to requests with, "Well, I really can't do that because I need to do X for my kids" or "I need to be free to do this for my son/my daughter, so I can't do that." I now realize that I often used my children as a way of avoiding making a choice based on my own self-knowledge. I could avoid taking responsibility for my decisions. Often my Yes was not *my* Yes, my No was not *my* No. "I can't" avoided responsibility. "I will" or "will not" accepts that responsibility. A single woman reminded her friends who had been majoring in children that now as older women, "There is nobody between you and you."

At menopause, many of us are presented with decisions that involve caring for our bodies. They include such questions as

Who can I trust to work with me as a doctor or health
    professional?
Do I need a hysterectomy?
Am I a candidate for hormone replacement therapy?

There really is "nobody between you and you" when it comes to making these kinds of decisions. There are certainly many sources for information now and skilled people available to assist us. However, as managers of our own health care, the ultimate decisions are in our hands.

These decisions can evoke in us questions of value, priority, responsibility, and commitment:

Do I want quality of life or quantity?
What is most important to me as I look toward getting older?
How do I see myself living as I get older?
What are the risks to me and what are the benefits to me if
    I take this action?
Am I willing to commit my time and energy to caring for myself
    in this way?

We have the opportunity as we approach our menopause to pay attention to our living with these decisions related to our bodies, as well as decisions related to our life purpose. We need to draw on our own life experience and the well of shared experience to make choices from the place of our own deep inner knowing. The group of women who named this kind of knowing *the sacred Know* described it from their own experience:

It is a different kind of knowing. A new way. Even though I have memory loss of detail, I have a clarity of knowing.

The sacred Know is a place of knowing the whole, even while we are in a place of brokenness.

The Crone, or Old Wise Woman, knows in a way that sees beyond vision. It's not that we're crazy. It's just tapping into intuition.

It is a maturing — being able to relax dependency on other kinds of knowing. You know it when you get in touch with it. It doesn't just come from the heart. It is a knowing that comes from the womb. I am feeling it more and more.

I love getting older! I love the knowingness. What I like is having the confidence — knowing and trusting myself, my feelings and my timing.

I am drawing on a deeper level of knowing. It is a body knowing, and my body doesn't lie. Being connected this way enables listening to myself and others. I affirm what I know as I trust my own experience.

The life passage of menopause allows us time to do some ingathering or harvesting of the fruits of our own experience. Remembering can be a part of this and a form of inner preparation for the second half of our lives. Remembering times of choice, turning points, small victories that were important to us in our growth is a part of this harvesting. There may also have been moments of fullness, perhaps only brief, in which we felt a sense of being fully alive. In recalling these, we touch an awareness of our gifts and abilities being used in a way that feels full. These moments in time are fruits of our harvest. They contain the seeds of new fruits.

We also have the opportunity, at this time of ingathering, to remember and to include experiences that may have been fearful, painful, and scarring. Yet they have gone into the harvest of all that has been. It is my experience, and I have learned from others, that at the core of these experiences is the potential for seeds of new self-expression and of wisdom. The seeds contained in these fruits can be shared and planted for the generations to come.

Henri Nouwen, author of many books on the spiritual life, speaks about fruitfulness from his own pilgrimage. *Lifesigns*, his recent book on "Intimacy, Fecundity, and Ecstasy in Christian Perspective," came out of his experience of living in the l'Arche community in France. Among his teachers were some severely handicapped people. From them he learned about "fecundity" or fruitfulness, and he learned about joy. The atmosphere in which he lived showed him by contrast how much our fear-dominated society does not foster that kind of lifefulness: "When fear dominates our lives, we cannot quietly and patiently protect the holy space where fruit can grow. . . . Sterility is one of the most obvious responses to fear. . . . [It is] the experience of not being truly alive, and therefore of being unable to give life."[3]

Nouwen suggests that fear of sterility or barrenness often pushes us to "frantic productivity." This awareness has been very helpful to me as I approach the end of my physical fertility:

> A product is something we make. . . . In our contemporary society, with its emphasis on accomplishment and success, we often live as if being productive is the same as being fruitful. Productivity gives us a certain notoriety and helps take away our fear of being useless. . . . The great mystery of fecundity is that it becomes visible when we have given up our attempts to control life and take the risk to let life reveal its own inner movements. Whenever we trust and surrender ourselves to the God of love, fruits will grow. Fruits can only come forth from the ground of intimate love. They are not made, nor are they the result of specific human actions that can be repeated. Neither predictable or definable, fruits are gifts to be received.[4]

I have been moved by women who are now expressing their growing sense of the richness of this time of life. Recently an older divorced woman, who has struggled economically, shared her experience of fruitfulness with a group. She told us of a recent "reunion" with her two grown sons and her ex-husband. She shared her sense of having given in that situation from the fruits of her life. "I was able to speak from all that I have gathered over the years, everything I have. And I am very grateful for these gifts. I feel great joy."

Fruits are blessings from a harvest of living. As we claim both the fruits that have grown through pain and those that have grown in moments of fullness, we are preparing the soil for a new season of fruitfulness.

9. Crossing the Threshold

"It is a threshold time!" said a woman whose menopause was recently celebrated. As she shared some of her thoughts and learnings with the small group who had gathered in her honor, we realized that it was from her own sacred Know that she named this time of life a threshold time.

As she explored this theme, we were reminded of a version of the Demeter myth in which a third goddess appears. Hecate (or Hekate), known for her connection with the underworld, is also the goddess of crossroads (she looks three ways) and of thresholds.

In this version of the familiar mother-maiden myth, Hecate, the elder wise woman, witnessed Persephone's descent into the underworld. She also was the one who guided her back to earth by lighting her way with a lamp. The three goddesses in this myth together represent aspects of the Great Goddess, the oldest godhead:

> According to ancient tradition, the Great Goddess was
> always triple. Her triplicity is seen in the waxing moon, the
> full moon, and the waning moon, and in how she ruled the
> world and underworld. In human terms she was Maiden,
> Mother, and Crone. It is these major phases of a woman's
> life . . . that are encompassed by the Demeter story.[1]

Those of us who are entering the third phase of our life cycle may
find it helpful to become acquainted with this goddess of the waning
moon. As crone or elder wise woman, Hecate was known as "the
goddess whom Zeus honors above all . . . a great mother goddess
associated with fair judgment and with victory in battle and game,
with the fruitfulness of the sea, the flocks, and the human family."[2]

Hecate's association with fruitfulness connected her with
Demeter, the mother. Her knowledge of the underworld connected
her with Persephone, the maiden, whom she assisted in her passage
to and from that encounter with the depths. It is her light that led
Persephone in her return and thus in the return of new life to the
earth. "Awesome are her skills but always Hekate taught the same
lesson: Without death there is no life."[3] She is a powerful figure for
those of us learning about letting go at this time in our lives.

The elder wise woman's power is represented by the waning
moon, which is a part of the moon's on-going cycle, as letting go is
part of the relational cycle. Those of us who are willing to explore the
spiritual movement of letting go, which *is* a form of death, will also
be able to embrace the passage of menopause as a movement into new
life in the final third of our life cycle. We have the opportunity to make
our peace with Hecate as an aspect of the feminine life rhythm and as
an aspect of our own life experience.

The word *crone* conjures up unpleasant images for many of us.
Its derivation is from the root word meaning "carrion" or "carcass,"
a strong and graphic image of our fears about this third phase of our
lives. However, as with many aspects of this life passage, we have the
power to create our own experience and to name it.

The imagery suggested by Hecate, the crone, may speak deeply
to some of us. One woman reflecting on the derivation of the word

had this insight: "The natural rhythm of decomposition and recomposition is suggested by the word 'crone.' With decomposition the beauty shines through. At this time in our life we look better and better. We look like individuals . . . beauty is transformed." In speaking of the life passage of menopause, another mid-life woman said, "I think we will find the Crone when we walk through that door."

Others may find this imagery a stumbling block, or it just may not speak to their experience. What is important for us, as we cross the threshold of this life passage, is being open to images that do touch our personal experience, for it is often these personal images that lead us on in our pilgrimage. The purpose of a pilgrimage, in Jean Shinoda Bolen's words, is to "quicken the Divine" in the pilgrim,[4] moving us toward an expression of our own true being. A pilgrimage often leads a person over territory that has been traveled by others. However, its significance to each pilgrim comes when she or he claims it as their own.

In the early days of bodily changes that pointed toward my coming menopause, a dream presented an image or symbol that has held rich meaning for me. Two apparent opposites were brought together and the paradox of that symbol caught my attention. The impact from that image actually moved me in the direction of exploring what women know about menopause:

I am in a gathering place with lots of children around. Some man is talking, and he refers to the feminine as "zero fruit." I feel a strong reaction to those words but hold back on saying anything.

As the words "zero fruit" are spoken by the male voice, I hear a negative overtone, and I see this symbol O. My attention is drawn to it. I have a very positive sense that it holds great potential, contrary to the way in which it is presented. Yet I feel sad because I realize that I know a great deal about "the feminine" experience and I hold back on what I know.

On waking I recorded the dream and my feelings in my journal: "It feels like either men know something that I don't, or I know something that they don't. Woke feeling they don't understand the feminine principle of receptivity, waiting, and darkness. Feel sad about that and somewhat alone." My conscious daytime self was still buying into the negative cultural myths of the menopausal woman and her zero fruit. My dreaming self, my deep self, however, knew much more about the inner movement of creative potential within the experience of menopause.

I let the dream symbol unfold over time. Its marvel for me was the paradox of zero, the ultimate emptiness, and fruit, the ultimate fullness. In the darkness of dreaming I sensed the interplay between these opposites. Later as I worked with the dream, I explored the word "zero." One definition was "a mathematical value intermediate between positive and negative values." I began to play with zero as a place of no value or judgment. Zero became empty space. Its connection with the word "fruit" in my dream gave that emptiness a sense of creative potential. It was this paradox that held energy for me. It led me to explore menopause with others.

The image of zero fruit came from a place of deep knowing in me, and it encouraged me to trust that in myself and in other women. We *do* know a lot about this particular aspect of the feminine life cycle. We also have a real understanding of paradox in our lives. This holding together of what often feels like two very different realities is the essence of feminine wisdom, according to Ann Belford Ulanov: "'Feminine wisdom' . . . is paradoxical wisdom which never juxtaposes opposites into 'either-or' pairs but gathers them into 'both-and' relationships."[5]

Around menopause many of us experience both a sense of physical limitation, the feeling of not being in control of our own bodies, and a sense of urgency about really living our lives. "I don't want to waste my time," one forty-nine-year-old woman said emphatically. "I want to get on with it!" Many women at this age express a strong desire to contribute and to make their lives count. This comes up in their concerns:

I have regrets about my use of time in the past.

I worry about a "calling" or a sense of professional productivity.

I have a sense of time urgency!

Our feminine wisdom calls us to embrace both our strong desire to live our lives meaningfully and our physical limitations, those intimations of our own mortality. By allowing both aspects of the truth of our experience to be so, we can begin to learn about pacing ourselves.

Pacing is new for many of us. We have been able to push our bodies and make them serve the many driving needs of our lives. Often our dreams will inform us that this is no longer working. A forty-seven-year-old woman recalled just such a dream: "I am pedaling down a freeway on a tricycle . . . feeling panicked as I pedal away, desperately trying to keep going."

A woman who works outside her home and is active in the community described her experience. She is approaching her menopause while being the mother of a young child as well as of teenagers:

I have what I call emotional blackouts. I am driving down the road, and I become aware that I have no idea where I'm going or what I'm supposed to be doing. I'm on overload. My life feels like mercury that has spilled on the floor. I keep trying to pick it up, and I just can't get it together. I'm tending to everybody else, and I don't know how to care for myself.

Many women approaching menopause have been mothering or nurturing others for a number of years. In *Ourselves, Growing Older*, the writers of the chapter on menopause point out that few of us, however, really know much about self-care. "New feminist research shows that many women learn to care for others first and only later to care for themselves."[6]

Learning how to care for ourselves does not come easily. We may not get the message until our bodies become our teachers and slow us down to a pace that gets our attention. Going with the limitations of our bodies — be they hot flashes, unpredictable flows, backaches, vaginal dryness, memory loss, or whatever — does call for changes in our lifestyles. We can learn to make choices about responding to those limitations. We *can* learn to care for ourselves.

Edith Sullwold, a mentor of mine, was remembering the years around her menopause. She shared with me her experience of hot flashes and the loss of energy. After going to a doctor whose prescription for estrogen she questioned, Edith began to reflect on her physical signs of change. She looked at her hot flashes as "the other end of all that fire that happened to create sexuality." She saw both as signs of the transformation process, beginning with the "natural shift and initiation from non-sexuality to sexuality." "The other end" was signaled by hot flashes that "acted as small transformers to a profound spiritual reality."

> I no longer wanted to get the energy back (as the doctor claimed estrogen would do). I realized that energy takes on a different quality. Now it's more like lighthouse energy: being very alive to observing yourself and others; active in a different way. Life is continuous. This is just the other end of transformation.

One aspect of that transformation was given a name by a woman who was part of a group that met regularly to explore their experience of menopause: "Maybe I am beginning to reap the benefits of all my mothering. All this practice at mothering, maybe we get the best of it after we've learned so much by trial and error. I can make a choice now to use my mothering energy for myself." As this mother of three adult daughters realized, we can reap the benefits of all our mothering when we choose to apply our skills to self-care. For those who still have young children and yet are ending their time of physical fertility with menopause, the experience of pregnancy can be instructive.

Pregnancy brings us to ourselves through our awareness of the changes in our body. The time of gestation is a preparatory time. No matter what we want to do, no matter how much we want to feel "in control," our body leads us. We often have to let go of well-made plans, tuning in to our bodily needs and responding in self-caring ways. Our mothering energy needs to be used first toward ourselves as we prepare to bring forth life.

The need for this kind of mothering energy is equally true during the longer preparatory time surrounding menopause. A single mother of a young child, reflecting on this idea, made the following comment: "At first I thought how can I mother myself during this passage when I still have a child to mother. Then I realized that I can be both mother to myself and to my son. Actually, caring for myself will enable me to have more to give him."

Mothering energy — strong, creative, compassionate, encouraging energy — is also needed as we engage in being mid-wife to our own expressions of new life during the passage of menopause. "We are giving birth to ourselves," a friend of mine said. And so it is for many women during this life passage. We move into a new form of self-expression.

Our sisters who have not borne children may have made their way through this doorway long before those of us for whom mothering has been our major self-identification. They may have discovered in their own experience what our Native American sisters have to teach about creation:

> Central to Keres theology [that of the Keres Indians of Laguna Pueblo] is the basic idea of the Creatrix as She Who Thinks rather than She Who Bears, of woman as creation thinker and female thought as origin of material and nonmaterial reality. In this epistemology, the perception of female power as confined to maternity is a limit on the power inherent in femininity.[7]

This understanding of woman as creation thinker gives a more inclusive scope to woman's potential for self-expression through the process of vitalizing and giving birth to our selves.

Often our unconscious leads us to this awareness through our dreams. Many women during the time surrounding menopause find themselves having dreams about babies. It is not unusual to have daytime concerns about being pregnant, given the irregularity of periods. Our unconscious may be dealing with that anxiety to some degree. But I believe that there is a deeper level of wisdom being expressed to us from our dreaming self, a statement of what is so.

We are at this life juncture, clearly moving toward infertility and yet having dreams about our potential for creating new life. Feminine wisdom *can* embrace this paradox. It "may well not be easy or comfortable." Esther De Waal uses these words to describe that very process in her book, *Living with Contradiction*:

> For as we learn to live with paradox, we have to admit that two realities can be equally true; we may be asked to hold together contrasting forces. The closer we come to something worthwhile, the more likely it is that paradox will be the only way to express it. The mind will never apprehend the truth of paradox. Only the heart can do that.[8]

The closer we come to understanding this with our hearts and to owning our feminine wisdom, the more exciting the possibilities become for us. As De Waal says, "This polarity, this holding together of opposites, this living with contradictions, presents us not with a closed system but a series of open doors."[9] This *is* a threshold time!

10. Joining the Community of Our Elders

O ur culture has not recognized the life passage surrounding menopause. Menopause is unlike the beginning of menstruation, which occurs at a known point in time. Climacteric, the whole process surrounding menopause, happens over several years. Yet both these bodily changes are crucial events in a woman's transformation process. As such, they need to be marked and recognized. Women are beginning to do this by creating their own rituals.

In one group, which had been meeting over a two-year period, a simple ceremony came into being when one woman recognized that her menses had ceased. It had been more than a year since her last menstrual flow, and she told the group that she would like to mark this passage. At their next gathering, this recognition took place. The group asked her to prepare to tell them of the wisdom that she had gained in these years, to speak of what she had learned. She took time with herself; the others prepared an empty space in the circle where they all sat. In the center of the circle was a stone that the woman had brought.

When the woman whose life passage was being celebrated entered the room, she claimed the empty space as the place of wisdom by sitting there. Holding the stone that represented where she was in her life, she slowly began to share what she had learned, her wisdom. Then each woman in turn spoke of what they had learned from her. Some gave her symbols of encouragement for her continued journey. Some spoke of their relationship with her. Others offered words of gratitude for what she had given them. It was a simple ceremony of recognition, celebration, and gratitude.

As we actively choose to engage in changing, we experience a transformation of life energy. According to Native American tradition, transformation of energy is the essence of ritual. Seen as a deeply feminine process, ritual is called "the power of mothering" in the Great Mother societies. "Ritual . . . means transforming something from one state or condition to another, and that ability is inherent in the action of mothering." It is "not so much the power to give birth . . . but the power to make, to create, to transform."[1]

Women who have come together to explore the unknown of the life passage of menopause have discovered that this shared experience can itself hold the quality of ritual. One woman, describing this feminine process, offered her insight. We encourage each other, she said, in "becoming more of who we already are. . . . That's the transformation process." As women, individually and together, we share the power to make, create, and transform.

In early Greek culture there were symbols for the transformation process from young girl to elder woman. The maiden was represented by the flower, and the mother by the fruit. The crone or elder wise woman, in the third phase of life, was represented by the seed: a powerful sign of death and new life. In that culture when the mother lost her fruitbearing ability, she entered the spiritual community of elders, the guardians of the mystery, death.

Given our life expectancy, we are actually moving from a phase of fruitbearing to the "second half of our life," as Sadja Greenwood has named it. This life season of autumn becomes a time of harvest, an ingathering of fruits that contain seeds of *new* fruitfulness for ourselves and generations to come.

These seeds are often discovered as we join the community of elder women and claim our own time of "generativity." This stage of life, so named by Erik Erikson, is presented as a time for "establishing and guiding the next generation."[2] Many of us in this time of ingathering look at our lives and reflect on the legacy that we are leaving for the generations to come. The concept of "generativity" is being expanded by women. Along with "establishing and guiding" generations to come, older women are challenging the outdated structures that have choked life.

Betty Friedan spoke recently to a gathering of women of many ages about the *new* feminine mystique, a mystique held in this country that women have a choice: either you work or you stay at home. In truth only a minority of women have this choice. "The issue is not either/or, but the personhood of women," says Friedan. Because our country has no national policy of child care or parental leave, the majority of women do not have the option to stay home with their children. It is economically impossible. Friedan's passion to establish laws and to create structures to give all women "real choices"[3] is her expression of generativity.

Those of us who have had the opportunity to make life choices are encouraged by some of our elders to reflect on those fruits of our lives thus far and to invest our life experience, our skills, and abilities in our own ways so that generations to come may live more fully. A woman who made the choice not to have children spoke of the legacy that she as an elder woman anticipates giving to others: "What we have to give back to life is not a child. I know I have something to give. I know I'm responsible to nurture it, feed it, house it, and bring it up for the next thirty years, and give it my time."

An essential part of the legacy we leave is our spiritual tradition. Maria Harris, in her book *Dance of the Spirit*, sees tradition not as something static, a thing to be handed down, but as dynamic and alive. "Tradition is the process by which humans communicate *ways* of knowing, *ways* of being, and *ways* of doing from one generation to the next. . . . Traditioning becomes the movements of handing on this life.[4] "Traditioning" has been one of the gifts of elder women. We become part of the transformation process for our younger sisters when we share our ways of knowing, being, and doing. We can offer a connection to the Source of Life and to the on-going feminine process that is being realized in their lives uniquely.

Often this kind of sharing begins to happen in subtle ways. During my thirties and early forties, I sought out many learning experiences by attending workshops, getting training, taking courses. I covered a lot of territory — literally in travel and figuratively in exposure to other people, their ideas, and their ways of doing things. As I began to approach menopause, I became aware that I was spending more time assimilating my own experience. For instance, instead of taking a workshop on menopause, I decided to create one with other women. Trusting the challenge of my "zero fruit" dream, I began to claim that I and we together know a lot about the feminine principle of receptivity, waiting, and darkness. Sharing this with younger women as a form of "traditioning" and spending time talking with older women has been my gradual way of joining the community of elders.

When we recognize ourselves as elder women, we open to a deeper sense of our own mortality. "Death seems less remote," as Connie Batten comments in her article entitled "Menopause: A Journey Homeward":

> When we are in the midst of the changes that signal the onset of menopause, death seems much less remote. This gives us a rare opportunity to see beyond our small ego-centered world. We can feel from a source deep within ourselves, the wonderful rightness of the more cyclical nature of the universe, and we can feel more directly than usual an awe and gratitude that we happen to be here to experience it. The fabric of our illusion rips and tears. We cannot help but see through it. We catch a glimpse of the Goddess without her veil. I feel myself pulled back, begin-

ning to remember something I once knew but had forgotten. It is not entirely comforting, but it is deeply true. Experiencing that truth, I feel substantial joy.[5]

Experiencing the truth of our mortality, we discover a longing to be truly alive — to experience the whole spectrum of life. Opening ourselves to our mortality, we also can know deep joy. As we embrace this paradox, we experience our feminine wisdom.

When we begin to share that wisdom, we join the community of elder women. This community is available to each one of us. We discover this as we begin talking with, listening to, reading about women who have lived longer than we have, our elders. We actually join that community when we begin to share our own experience with them. There is great support and encouragement for new life in this connection.

One woman became aware of her need for this community when she both discovered new life at the age of fifty-five and at the same time went through the death of her husband:

As a youngster I was an awkward tomboy and even more awkward as a teenager. Like the ugly duckling, I didn't know who I was. I tried to be like others for many years, but it didn't work. By the time I went to graduate school, I reached the point of recognizing what was true for me. I finally came into what I am meant to be. It came together for me in my mid-fifties.

In a course we were asked to find our own fairy tale. Then we were to retell it from the point of view of whatever character we chose. "The Ugly Duckling" was the one I chose, and the image of the swan became very powerful for me. Embodied in the image of the swan was beauty and grace. At the same time there was great power and strength. I have seen a female swan guarding the nest. Such beauty and ferocity, such strength as a protector. It is not just a pretty bird. Yet they are so beautiful in flight and in the water.

I came to see that one did not need to give up beauty and grace for strength and power. They are all there in the swan. Women are so often afraid of that. My husband understood this. For my birthday, he gave me a card that he had made, a collage of swan pictures. It was such an affirmation of the whole experience for me.

Within a year's time, he got sick and was dying. It took great courage for me to go ahead with school during that time. I drew on what felt like the swan's strength to do it. When he died ten years ago, I really changed. It was like *Swan Lake*. I was the grieving swan.

I am still greatly moved when I see a swan, especially in flight. That is rare. I've only seen one a couple of times. When I see it, a certain sadness is touched as I feel the loss of the great support that my husband gave me for my flight.

The sense of strength in flight of that time is not with me, but the image is still powerful. When I see a swan, there is that connection. Now when I see a solitary swan, that swan makes its own statement to me. That is the part that touches me now.

This woman's pilgrimage through grief has opened her to share what she has learned with other women:

It is important to know who you are and not get caught in the agenda of others. That is not to say other people's agendas don't have merit. But you become aware of your own mortality and the preciousness of time. You learn to harvest your time, winnowing out what is other people's stuff. Your choices can come much more from your essence.

Sharing our experience with others helps us name it and claim that which is ours. This can happen with people who are newly in our lives because of shared experience, such as widowhood. It can also happen with people from our past. Being with people who know how to listen makes all the difference.

A small group of women who lived together for four years while in college came together for two days in a mountain retreat. The purpose of this gathering was to reconnect after twenty-five years of separation. We decided to give each other one hour of time to tell our stories in whatever way we chose to do so. As each woman took her turn, the rest of us listened with only an occasional question for clarification. It was an opportunity for each person to be heard with that kind of listening that enables the speaker to make discoveries while she speaks. There were tears, great laughter, moments of healing and deeper understanding. There was celebration of the harvest of who we were and who we are becoming both as individuals and as a group. We were together becoming a community of elders.

We can also create our community by linking together many separate individuals whose lives touch us, challenge us, encourage us on our way. One woman now approaching fifty recalled a simple encouraging conversation with an older friend: "I was speaking about my life. She said to me, 'If you think forty is great, just wait 'til you are sixty.'" Our community of elders may extend beyond friends or relatives. It may include authors, poets, artists, political activists, public figures, fictional or historic persons. The community comes into being through our own sense of connection.

Marion Wright Edelman, founder, president, and spokesperson for the Children's Defense Fund, is part of my community of elders, even though she is a year younger than I and we have never met. Her lifework as an advocate for children and her early sense of generativity touch and challenge me now at this time in my life:

> Service was as much a part of my upbringing as eating breakfast and going to school. . . . It was clear that it was the very purpose of life. In that context, you're not obligated to win. You are obligated to keep trying, to keep doing the best you can every day. Helping others had the highest value. There was no black home for the aged in South Carolina when I was growing up, so my daddy, who was a minister,

started one across the street, and we all had to get out there and cook and serve. My mother died a few years ago, still running that home for the aged. She was cooking for six old people, all of them younger than she was.[6]

As she describes her own work through the Children's Defense Fund, Edelman speaks of the legacy that she wants to leave for generations of children to come:

Our goal is to show the nation that preventive investment in kids has got to become the cornerstone of American domestic policy. . . . What I want to do is to see that this country feeds hungry kids. The legacy that I want to leave is a child-care system that says that no kid is going to be left alone or left unsafe.[6]

These words appeared with Edelman's black-and-white portrait in the powerful photographic exhibit called *I Dream a World: Portraits of Black Women Who Changed America*.

A seventy-year-old friend of mine, who is a gifted cabinetmaker, shared with me Daisy Newman's reflections "On Turning Seventy." Newman's words named my friend's experience also:

If you are an artist with enough to live on and (overlooking a twinge or two) in fair health, it's a rewarding age. You've served your apprenticeship. There's no need to compete, to prove yourself. The bliss of creating is always yours, yet something new is stirring in you: a secret knowledge, an intimation, waiting to be revealed in your work. Why couldn't it have come sooner?

All those years had to be used up first, crammed with experience, joys, and sorrows. . . .

You're free now to pour out your whole essence, just as, at sugaring time in Vermont, you used to pour maple syrup over the family's pancakes. It took gallons of sap, piles of cordwood, and hours of boiling on the back of that superannuated stove to produce enough syrup for a single breakfast, yet you poured it with loving abandon — the whole distillation of your labors.

No, it won't last long. Nevertheless, it's a beautiful time, a time of value, even promise.[7]

The experience of an elder feeling free to pour out her essence is a wonderful promise for those of us approaching our menopause and our entry into the community of elders.

The pouring out of one's essence names for me the sense I have when I hear a bird sing its song. Early one morning in June I was waking but still in semi-sleep, aware that I needed to come up with an imaging experience for the "menopause group," meeting that morning. I was, perhaps, in a state of openness. All at once I heard the clearest bird call right outside my window. Simultaneously words came from somewhere deep within. I heard them as clearly as I heard the song outside my window: "I want to write a book."

Rising then, the inner song sounded through my meditation and group-planning time. I continued to hear the words, "I want to write a book." I wrote in my journal:

No more a mocking bird
    yet I have learned so much
        from all my teachers
    their intention however
        was never
        that I should sing their song.

Sing your own song
    I hear in this morning's bird call
        filling up the sky
            with liquid laughter sound.

Oh, yes, I do want to and will
    beginning now, today . . .
    and I say thank you to you

unnamed bird
song bird
my-own-song-bird.

A friend of mine who knows birds well told me that to her a bird's song is the bird's "I am!" statement. I loved that. It is the bird announcing the presence of itself, its particular territory, its "I am!" for all the world to hear.

Elizabeth Dodson Gray, editor of *Sacred Dimensions of Women's Experience*, wrote the final article in that book, entitled "Why Do Birds Sing? Healing After Trauma." Awaking on a "morning cool enough to subdue my hot flashes," after a long, slow process of healing from a physical trauma, she reflected,

> This was the first morning in two-and-a-half years when I was not in pain. I was reveling in my newly regained abilities to feel totally sensual and be without pain, when I noticed the birds singing. . . . Listening to the birds through my open bedroom window, I again felt as though I were somehow slipping late into a pew and joining a celebration already in progress. But this time I asked myself a new question — "Why do the birds sing?" The answer came to me strong and clear from someplace deep in me or deep within the universe — "Birds sing because rejoicing is the center of the universe."[8]

For me those words made a deep connection, for one of the questions of my soul has been "How can I express joy when there is so much pain and suffering?" Gray's words come from a pilgrimage through suffering. She speaks of joy as the center and rejoicing as "the flow of Being in the universe."

In my own pilgrimage, a very slow and quiet journey, I am still coming to recognize that the deep flowing River of Living Water that has nourished my life and all creation includes the tears of great sorrow and deep joy. It is this underground stream that feeds our souls and, in Mystery, is also the source of our true being. Claiming our oneness with this source, drawing on it for the replenishment of our being, we can continue our pilgrimage through menopause with a sense of joy.

We can also celebrate with our elders the rich harvest of life's fruits. Those grown in pain and those grown through moments of fullness can be used to nurture, feed, and transform energy for our selves, our loved ones, and our world. This shared abundance makes it possible in the autumn time of our lives to celebrate with thanksgiving.

Notes

Preface

1. John Sharkey, *Celtic Mysteries: The Ancient Religion* (New York: Thames and Hudson, 1987), 7.
2. Ibid., 72–73.
3. Elizabeth Dodson Gray, *Sacred Dimensions of Women's Experience* (Wellesley, Massachusetts: Roundtable Press, 1988), 241.

1. Trusting Our Experience

1. Robert A. Wilson, *Feminine Forever* (New York: M. Evans and Company, Inc., 1966), chapter 5.
2. Jane Fonda, *Women Coming of Age* (New York: Simon & Schuster, 1984), 117.
3. Winnifred Berg Cutler, Celso-Ramon Garcia, and David A. Edwards, *Menopause: A Guide for Women and the Men Who Love Them* (New York: W. W. Norton & Company, 1983), 31.

2. Sharing Our Experience

1. Christine Downing, *Journey Through Menopause: A Personal Rite of Passage* (New York: Crossroad, 1987), 10.
2. Anne Cameron, *Daughters of Copper Woman* (Vancouver: Press Gang Publishers, 1981), 27.
3. Ibid., 61-62.
4. Paula Gunn Allen, *The Sacred Hoop: Recovering the Feminine in American Indian Traditions* (Boston: Beacon Press, 1986), 28.
5. Matthew Fox, *Original Blessing* (Sante Fe: Bear & Company, 1983).
6. Elisabeth Kubler-Ross, *On Death and Dying* (New York: Macmillan, 1969).
7. Downing, *Journey Through Menopause*, 25.
8. Irene P. Stiver and Jean Baker Miller, "From Depression to Sadness in Women's Psychotherapy," *Work in Progress*, Stone Center Working Papers Series, No. 36 (Wellesley, Massachusetts: Wellesley College, 1988), 1.

3. Renaming Our Experience

1. Winnifred Cutler, et al., *Menopause: A Guide for Women and the Men Who Love Them* (New York: W. W. Norton & Company, 1983), 47.
2. Christine Downing, *Journey Through Menopause* (New York: Crossroad, 1987), 25-26.
3. Paula Gunn Allen, *The Sacred Hoop* (Boston: Beacon Press, 1986), 13.
4. Ibid., 14.
5. Ibid., 22.
6. Jean Shinoda Bolen, "Women's Spirituality," Interface Workshop (Watertown, Massachusetts, January 1988). Bolen has developed her thoughts on menopause more fully in a tape titled *Wise Woman Archetype: Menopause as Initiation* (1991), available from Sounds True Recordings, 735 Walnut Street, Boulder, Colorado, 80302.

4. Remembering

1. Carol Christ, *Diving Deep and Surfacing: Women Writers on Spiritual Quest* (Boston: Beacon Press, 1980), 5.
2. Paula Gunn Allen, *The Sacred Hoop* (Boston: Beacon Press, 1986), 11.
3. Nelle Morton, *The Journey Is Home* (Boston: Beacon Press, 1985), 127.
4. Eugene Gendlin, *Focusing* (New York: Bantam Books, 1981), 8.

5. Peter A. Campbell and Edwin M. McMahon, *Bio-Spirituality: Focusing as a Way to Grow* (Chicago: Loyola University Press, 1985), chapter 2. This is the best resource on applying the "Focusing" technique.

5. Grieving Our Losses

1. Marge Piercy, "Something to look forward to," *Available Light* (New York: Alfred A. Knopf, 1988), as quoted in *Women of the 14th Moon: Writings on Menopause*, ed. by Dena Taylor and Amber Coverdale Sumrall (Freedom, California: The Crossing Press, 1991), 13.
2. Elisabeth Kubler-Ross, *On Death and Dying* (New York: Macmillan, 1969).
3. This was the slogan on an Extraderm information kit, produced by CIBA Pharmaceutical Company, Summit, New Jersey.
4. Irene P. Stiver and Jean Baker Miller, "From Depression to Sadness in Women's Psychotherapy," *Work in Progress*, Stone Center Working Papers Series, No. 36 (Wellesley, Massachusetts: Wellesley College, 1988), 1.
5. Ibid., 5.
6. Christine Downing, *Journey Through Menopause* (New York: Crossroad, 1987), 119, citing Joseph Campbell.

6. Allowing Empty Space

1. Judith Duerk, *Circle of Stones: A Woman's Journey to Herself* (San Diego: LuraMedia, 1989), 58.
2. R. Cameron Borton, "How to Meditate" (Unpublished monograph, 1989).
3. Annie Dillard, *Teaching a Stone to Talk: Expeditions and Encounters* (New York: Harper & Row, 1982), 47.
4. Ibid., 48.

7. Letting Go . . . to Embrace

1. Charlene Spretnak, *Lost Goddesses of Early Greece: A Collection of Pre-Hellenic Myths* (Boston: Beacon Press, 1984), 114.
2. Adrienne Rich, *Of Woman Born* (New York: W. W. Norton, 1976), 226.
3. Aurora Levins Morales and Rosario Morales, *Getting Home Alive* (Ithaca: New York: Firebrand Books, 1986), Introduction.

4. Janet Surrey, "The Mother-Daughter Relationship: Themes in Psycho-therapy," tape (Wellesley, Massachusetts: Wellesley College Stone Center, 1989).
5. Janice Mirikitani, "For My Daughter," the dedication of "Sing With Your Body," as quoted by Tillie Olsen in *Mother to Daughter, Daughter to Mother* (New York: The Feminist Press, 1984), 7. The poem was originally published in *Awake in the River* (Isthmus Press, 1978).

8. Knowing and Choosing

1. Frederick Nietzsche, *The Portable Nietzsche*, ed. by Walter Kaufmann (New York: Penguin Books, Viking Portable Library, 1977), 137.
2. Ibid., 138-39.
3. Henri J. M. Nouwen, *Lifesigns: Intimacy, Fecundity, and Ecstasy in Christian Perspective* (New York: Doubleday, 1986), 57.
4. Ibid., 60, 65-66.

9. Crossing the Threshold

1. Jennifer Barker Woolger and Roger J. Woolger, *The Goddess Within: A Guide to Eternal Myths That Shape Women's Lives* (New York: Fawcett-Columbine, 1989), 283.
2. Christine Downing, *Journey Through Menopause* (New York: Crossroad, 1987), 37.
3. Charlene Spretnak, *Lost Goddesses of Early Greece* (Boston: Beacon Press, 1984), 83.
4. Jean Shinoda Bolen, "Women's Spirituality," Interface Workshop (Watertown, Massachusetts, January 1988).
5. Ann Belford Ulanov, *The Feminine in Jungian Psychology and in Christian Theology* (Evanston, Illinois: Northwestern University Press, 1971), 208.
6. Paula Brown Doress and Diana Laskin Siegal, *Ourselves, Growing Older: Women Aging with Knowledge and Power* (New York: Simon and Schuster, 1987), 117.
7. Paula Gunn Allen, *The Sacred Hoop* (Boston: Beacon Press, 1986), 15.
8. Esther De Waal, *Living with Contradiction: Reflections on the Rule of St. Benedict* (London: Collins, 1989), 33-34.
9. Ibid., 32-33.

10. Joining the Community of Our Elders

1. Paula Gunn Allen, *The Sacred Hoop* (Boston: Beacon Press, 1986), 29.
2. Erik Erikson, *Childhood and Society,* 2nd ed. (New York: W. W. Norton & Co., 1963), 67.
3. Betty Friedan, "Real Choices: A New Feminine Mystique" (Northampton, Massachusetts: Smith College, lecture, June 1990).
4. Maria Harris, *Dance of the Spirit: The Seven Steps of Woman's Spirituality* (New York: Bantam Books, 1989), 147.
5. Connie Batten, "Menopause: A Journey Homeward," *Woman of Power* 14 (Summer 1989), 59.
6. Brian Lanker, *I Dream a World: Portraits of Black Women Who Changed America* (New York: Stewart, Tabori and Chang, 1989), 121.
7. Daisy Newman, *A Golden String* (New York: Harper & Row, 1987), 153.
8. Elizabeth Dodson Gray, ed., *Sacred Dimensions of Women's Experience* (Wellesley, Massachusetts: Roundtable Press, 1988), 241.

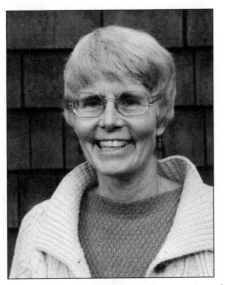

Joan C. Borton

J oan Borton began writ- ing in a journal at the same time that she was discovering the relationship between religion and psychology at Smith College. The connection between the three has led her along the way to her current work.

Joan is an early childhood specialist and consultant to parents, schools, and day-care centers. She also has a private counseling practice with women and children. Leading retreats and workshops with groups of women has provided her the opportunity to explore menopause as a life passage. She has contributed to *Women of the 14th Moon: Writings on Menopause* (Crossing Press) and *Readings in Psychosynthesis: Theory, Practice, and Process.*

She and her husband, Cam, a United Church of Christ minister, have three grown children: Jenni, Lawrie, and Jim.

LuraMedia Publications

BANKSON, MARJORY ZOET
Braided Streams: *Esther and a Woman's Way of Growing*
Seasons of Friendship: *Naomi and Ruth as a Pattern*

BOHLER, CAROLYN STAHL
Prayer on Wings: *A Search for Authentic Prayer*

BOZARTH, ALLA RENEE
Womanpriest: *A Personal Odyssey (Rev. Ed.)*

GEIGER, LURA JANE
Astonish Me, Yahweh Leader's Guide

and **PATRICIA BACKMAN**
Braided Streams Leader's Guide

and **SUSAN TOBIAS**
Seasons of Friendship Leader's Guide

and **SANDY LANDSTEDT, MARY GECKELER, PEGGIE OURY**
Astonish Me, Yahweh!: *A Bible Workbook-Journal*

JEVNE, RONNA FAY
It All Begins With Hope: *Patients, Caretakers, and the Bereaved Speak Out*

and **ALEXANDER LEVITAN**
No Time for Nonsense: *Getting Well Against the Odds*

KEIFFER, ANN
Gift of the Dark Angel: *A Woman's Journey through Depression toward Wholeness*

LODER, TED
Eavesdropping on the Echoes: *Voices from the Old Testament*
Guerrillas of Grace: *Prayers for the Battle*
No One But Us: *Personal Reflections on Public Sanctuary*
Tracks in the Straw: *Tales Spun from the Manger*
Wrestling the Light: *Ache and Awe in the Human-Divine Struggle*

LUCIANI, JOSEPH
Healing Your Habits: *Introducing Directed Imagination*

MCMAKIN, JACQUELINE
with **SONYA DYER**
Working from the Heart: *For Those Who Search for Meaning and Satisfaction in Their Work*

MEYER, RICHARD C.
One Anothering: *Biblical Building Blocks for Small Groups*

MILLETT, CRAIG
In God's Image: *Archetypes of Women in Scripture*

O'CONNOR, ELIZABETH
Search for Silence *(Revised Edition)*

RAFFA, JEAN BENEDICT
The Bridge to Wholeness: *A Feminine Alternative to the Hero Myth*

SAURO, JOAN
Whole Earth Meditation: *Ecology for the Spirit*

SCHAPER, DONNA
A Book of Common Power: *Narratives Against the Current*
Stripping Down: *The Art of Spiritual Restoration*

WEEMS, RENITA J.
Just a Sister Away: *A Womanist Vision of Women's Relationships in the Bible*

The Women's Series

BORTON, JOAN
Drawing from the Women's Well: *Reflections on the Life Passage of Menopause*

CARTLEDGE-HAYES, MARY
To Love Delilah: *Claiming the Women of the Bible*

DAHL, JUDY
River of Promise: *Two Women's Story of Love and Adoption*

DUERK, JUDITH
Circle of Stones: *Woman's Journey to Herself*

O'HALLORAN, SUSAN *and* **DELATTRE, SUSAN**
The Woman Who Lost Her Heart

RUPP, JOYCE
The Star in My Heart: *Experiencing Sophia, Inner Wisdom*

SCHAPER, DONNA
Superwoman Turns 40: *The Story of One Woman's Intentions to Grow Up*

LuraMedia, Inc. , 7060 Miramar Rd., Suite 104, San Diego, CA 92121
Books for Healing and Hope, Balance and Justice.